PREKSHA YOGA

MANAGEMENT FOR COMMON AILMENTS

PRESKSHA YOGA

MANAGEMENT FOR COMMON AILMENTS

Dr J. P. N.Mishra
Head
Department of Science of Living
Preksha Meditation and Yoga
Jain Vishva Bharati Institute (Deemed University)
Ladnun - 341306, Rajasthan (INDIA)

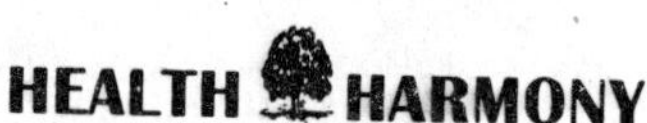

An imprint of
B. Jain Publishers (P) Ltd.
An ISO 9001 : 2000 Certified Company
USA — EUROPE — INDIA

Printed in India

First Edition : 1999
Reprint Edition: 2004, 2007

Published by:
B. Jain Publishers Pvt. Ltd
1921/10, Chuna Mandi, Pahar Ganj
New Delhi 110 055 (India) *Phones:* 2358 3100, 2358 1300

Printed at:
Unision Techno Financial Consultants Pvt. Ltd.
522, Patpar Ganj, Delhi-110092

BOOK CODE / ISBN: 978-81-319-0120-5

DEDICATED

To

My Dada Ji

and

My uncle Shri Lalta Prasad Ji Mishra,

who is my guru,

my teacher and my mentor.

ॐ नमः शिवाय

ॐ नमो भगवते वासुदेवाय

या देवी सर्वभूतेषु मातृरूपेण संस्थितां।
नमस्तस्यै नमस्तस्यै नमस्तस्यै नमो नमः।।

अरहंते शरणम् पवज्जामि, सिद्धे शरणम् पवज्जामि।
साहू शरणम् पवज्जामि, केवलि पण्णत्तम् धम्मम् शरणम् पवज्जामि।।

I burn my candle at both ends;
It may not last the night.
But oh! my friends, and ah! my foes;
It makes a lovely light.

science of disease and its treatment, whereas yoga is a science of health. Its techniques are based on most precise understanding of adequate and balanced functioning of both human body and mind, to achieve the state of good health, vitality and youthfulness in all conditions.

All human beings tend to attain the state of health and happiness, that too free from all pains and fears. That can be attained only by practising the method of *self training.* It (the self training) works through experience, and even after being very subtle, self training brings one to the optimal level of understanding about the significant factors involved in health and happiness. It has been found to be one of the best available therapy methods. Preksha Meditation is an effective technique of self training. It has been so designed that it helps each bodily cell to revitalize; it trains, cleans and relaxes ever wandering mind by realising the subconscious and unconscious mysteries; it strengthens the power of conscious reasoning control over the reactions to various external and internal stimuli; and it establishes firm control of the reasoning mind over the transformation of body chemistry en route the effective functioning of psycho-neuro-endocrine system.

In this manual of therapeutics I have tried to incorporate and explain various facets of yoga and preksha meditation therapy to manage a few of the commonly occurring diseases and disorders. The monograph has been divided in three section. Section I deals with the fundamentals of yoga and preksha meditation — their definition, philosophical basis, their relationship to the human health, both in normal condition and in the condition of disease, their therapeutic basis, and nutritional influence

From the Author's Desk

Human being is a combination of gross material structural organs, and subtle invisible element consciousness. Structural organs include various systems of the body, e.g. respiratory system, digestive system etc. and a few special senses life eyes, ear etc. Consciousness, mind and intellect are a few internal subtle and intangible ones, which constitute nonmaterial elements. Passions, feelings and emotions are the special characteristics associated with conscious mind, and are termed as primal drives. They are the prime movers of the three fold activities — mental, vocal and physical, to be manifested in gross physical body in association with external structural organs through an inter-communicating mechanism. The outcome of such manifestations is profound negative influence on and contamination of mental state. Decontaminating it to the goodness is the supreme aim of the science and art of the yoga and meditation.

In yoga philosophy too, physical body is stated to be only one aspect of health. Mind and spirit are the other components of the health and are given equal importance. There, it is mentioned that mind must heal for the body to mend; mind should remain healthy to keep up the physical health. In other words it may be inferred that yoga integrates the science of mind, body and spirit.

The natural state of body is health, where every smallest unit or part and its function has only one overriding biological aim — to seek and restore health at all time. The modern medicine largely looks like the on yogic therapy. In section II techniques of yogic exercises, asanas, pranayam, mudra and bandh, and preksha meditation have been elaborated in the mode of "proceed step-by-step". In section III, brief account of a few selected diseases (25) has been given, mentioning their causative factors and basic sysmptoms. This is being followed by a capsule therapy programme comprising the selected yogic exercises, asanas, pranayam, preksha and anupreksha, in the relevance to each disease separately.

I have tried my best to keep an effective but easy and workable approach to elaborate the subject matter. I look forward to hear from the inellectuals, experts and worldwide readership whatever related to the critical assessment of this write-up. That will help it to improve further.

Ladnun
August 10, 1999

J.P.N. Mishra

———— :::::::: ————

Acknowledgement

I am thankful to the almighty God, who blessed me with a healthy body, mind and spirit to serve. Further I owe my head with esteem reverence in the holiy feet of Ganadhipati Gurudev Tulsi and reverend H. H. Acharya Shri Mahaprajna, who not only admitted me as a scholar in the school of Yoga and Meditation, but also trained me to live a spiritual academic life. I will remain indebted for their blessings showered upon me. I am also grateful of Prof. Muni Shri Mahendra Kumar and Muni Shri Dharmesh Kumar for their kind motivation, inspiration and guidance every now and then.

I hereby bestow a special debt of gratitude to Prof. B. C. Lodha, Vice Chancellor, JVBI, Ladnun, who not only encouraged me to live like a scientist, to behave like a yogi, and to produce something extraordinary in academic field, but also provided all sorts of facilities in the institute of work.

I will be failing in my duty if I donot remember Dr. (Mrs.) Usha Sachdeva, Professor of Physiology, AIIMS, New Delhi, from whom I have learnt secrets of academic life. She is my real academic mentor. I am also grateful to Prof. R. L. Bijlani, Prof. V. Mohan Kumar and Dr. H. N. Mallick, from AIIMS, New Delhi, from whom I have picked up a lot in the field of physiology and yoga.

I am also thankful to my friend Dr. Birmal K. Chhajer, Director, SAAOL Heart Centre, New Delhi, and Swami Dharmanad, Director, Adhyatma Sadhana Kendra, New Delhi, who become instrumental in establishing me at J.V.B.I., Ladnun.

My special heart-felt thanks are due to Dr. B. R. Dugar, my senior colleague, for his continuous insistence to write something on the subject of Yoga and Preksha Meditation. I am also thankful to Dr. Anil Dhar and Dr. B. P. Gaur, my colleagues, who have always given their valuable advises like a friend and well wisher. I express my sincere thanks to my other colleagues Dr. J. R. Bhattacharya, Dr. H. S. Pandey, Dr. Jinendra Jain, Dr. Ashok Jain, Dr. A. P. Tripathi and Shri Ashutosh Pradhan, who were always very nice to me. It extend my heart-felt thanks to my elder brother and friend Dr. Gopalji Mishra whose company for mere two years gave me the pleasure beyond words. I also express my regards to Prof. Musafir Singh and Prof. Dayanand Bhargava. I am thankful to Shri Nepal P. Gang, Editor, 'Preksha Dhyan', for his cooperation in providing relevant literature many times.

I wish to express my real gratitude to Dr. B. L. Jain, my good friend and well wisher, whose elderly advices have encouraged me many a times to achieve new heights of success in my academic career and personal life.

I acknowledge my sincere thanks to my students Mr. Sanjeev Gupta and Mr. Abodh Srivastava, along with Ms. Mamta Mishra for their valuable contribution in terms of performing various exercises during photographic sessions. I am also thankful to Shri Jagdish Sharma of "Studio Chitra", Ladnun for preparing the photoprints so nicely.

My special thanks and regards goes to Shri Prem Nathji Jain, who honoured the manuscript of this book for publication. Without his sincere and willing efforts this publication would have not been possible.

I must extend my sincere thanks to all those who have contributed, by any means towards the substance and shape of this book.

Lastly, I wish I could find some words to express my heart-felt thanks to my wife Mrs. Vijai Mishra for her constant moral encouragement in building-up my enthusiasm, and her magnificent devotion to family despite her own professional liabilities. I am very sincerely thankful to my lovely daughter Mamta Mishra and son Ashutosh Mishra, from whom I have borrowed their own time of enjoyment for my academic work.

J. P. N. Mishra

———— :::::::: ————

Introduction

We are living in transient phase of continuously fast changing period. What we learn today, the same becomes obsolete day after tomorrow. Every one is running behind the materialistic world to catch hold of something big, but imaginary, that too in unplanned way. In this process sometimes we do achieve some thing, but in due course we leave aside our real 'ourselves'. And when we assess our achievements we find that we have paid very heavy price, for that illusory achievement, in terms of mental peace, physical health and spiritual self.

It is a bitter reality, without any dispute, that we cannot escape from the crazy race, up to certain extent, for external needs and desires, because we have to remain in that type of social set-up. But at the same time is not it our responsibility to be aware of extraordinary alarming pressure being exerted on our mind and body due to that crazy race? The pressure of modern life style, pressure of so called advanced knowledge of science and technology and the pressure of everchanging unstable thoughts have now gone beyond our capacity to bear, and that have led to an unproportionate growth of physical sickness and diseases, as well as psychosomatic disorders.

In today's so called modern society most of the people are suffer from various sophisticated and uncurable ailments which were not reported by ancient people. To stress, an overused phenomenon, has found a firm place in our New Age Vocabulary, just as fast food, junk bonds or software packages have. So, debased by misuse it generates only negativity in most people's minds. It plays havoc with the mind and body forcing them to revolt in myriad ways. It is believed that stress results from never ending desires and needs of an individual being greater than his actual capacity. In response to the threatening situation of stress stimulus several physiological changes take place in the body, which may be summarised as Fight-n-Fight reaction. Chronic stress both lowers resistance to illness and intensifies its impact. Often, there are recurrent patterns where illness coincides with stressful periods and may linger even after the stress is over. It is general belief that stress results in non-specific diseases, but recently there has been new thinking on the link between several serious diseases of almost uncurable nature and chronic disruption of immune responses because of repeated stress stimulation.

The question stands — is this 'stress devil' destined to be our life long companion? Do we have any option to escape it? The answer is — yes! We have the option, whose implementation will bring about changes in our life styles, in our thinking and in our conscious reasoning capacity. That will not only bring back the mental peace and joy but also yield the perfect state of physical, mental and emotional health. And that sacred mode of option is nothing but yoga and meditation.

The life of an individual is full of miscellaneous events and those events are responsible for variety of experiences and feelings. Those personal experiences cause either elevation or degeneration in the level of consciousness. In one individual it is in progressive state and in other, it is in the state of degeneration. However in some other direction of development the first group of individuals, with elevated level of consciousness, may lag behind, while the second group might have made considerable progress. All these ultimately affect the divine "self" which has uninterrupted flow of consciousness. This results in different levels of physical, mental, emotional and spiritual health. The foremost aim of yoga is to help us establish a perfect harmony among them and to obtain their optimal levels. Yoga is not only a theory and philosophy, but also it is an effective technology. As a philosophy, it guides us as to understand what is the ultimate truth and what should be our way of life. As a technology it helps us in choosing the right path. It has great therapeutic value too. The regular practice of yoga brings about peace of mind and mental equilibrium. The tranquility thus obtained bestows on its way a healthy mind in a healthy body free from disease, and this very concept has formed the basis of present write - up in your hand.

Eminent therapy specialists and general practitioners have now realised that meditation is a powerful therapy both for maintaining good health and for healing. Regular practice of meditation positively influences the central control mechanism which is responsible for the state of homeostasis in the body, leading to not only physical goodness but also psychical goodness, by eradicating all evils from one's thoughts, speech and action. Improvement of physical health and cure of serious illness without injurious drugs is one of the several valuable contributions of the meditation. Preksha meditation is one of the most comprehensive available meditation systems which helps the practitioner to achieve the goal of healthy body and healthy mind, by awakening and developing the conscious reasoning power along with control over irrational instincts.

Diet and life-style play a pivotal role in maintaining the sound health state. Diet comprising "Sattvic food" should always be preferred, as it not only claims to help promote longevity, health and happiness but also helps maintain a clear and unwavering mind. It should be wholesome, palatable and congenial to the body, and should not be eaten merely to gratify the senses. Although, in normal conditions, the balanced diet comprises all essential micro- and macronutrients in the standard quantity, in the state of disease the quantity of a particular nutrient/nutrients is to be changed proportionately to cope up with the requirement of healing process. This factor has been taken into account while prescribing/recommending the diet in case of a person suffering from a particular disease and undertaking Preksha-Yoga management programme.

Life style is another significant factor which affects the state of physical, mental and emotional health. Irrespective of the profession one has to adopt such a life-style which may bring about a balance in our thinking, doing and being. It should help us to regulate and restrict ourselves, our desires, our weaknesses and our sickness. Life style, in fact, is a composite phenomenon which includes way of thinking, way of doing, way of behaving, way of eating, way of sleeping, and so on. It should be of such type which makes us aware of all such activities and ourselves. This will help bring integration of the human health in all dimensions of human existence.

——————:::::::: ——————

ABOUT THE BOOK

Every person must be self-trained to maintain the body in perfectly sound health, by keeping it physically active, mentally at peace and protected from environmental influences. The book on preksha-yoga serves as an ideal guide by presenting methodical, illustrated details of yogic practice, proper nutrition, meditation etc. for management of common diseases in clear, simple language, written by an expert professor in human physiology well versed in yoga.

I sincerely hope that this book would keep our readers attain a healthy and happy life.

Dr. P. N. Jain
Publisher

CONTENTS

From the Author's Desk (v)

Acknowledgement (viii)

Introduction (xi)

SECTION I

Yoga, Preksha Meditation and Health **1-64**

- What is yoga 2
- Yoga philosophy 5
- Components of yoga 9
- Preksha meditation 28
- Yoga and health 37
- Therapeutic basis of yoga 43
- Therapeutic basis of preksha meditation 48
- Nutrition and yogic diet 53

SECTION II

Methodologies of Yoga and Preksha Meditation **65-163**

- Yogic exercises 66
- Shat kriyas 81
- Asanas 95
- Mudra and bandh 125
- Kayotsarga (relaxation) 135
- Pranayama 143
- Preksha meditation 155

SECTION III

Preaksha-Yogic Management of Common Diseases and Disorders (165-220)

- General precautions 166
- Headache 167
- Thyroid diseases 169
- Coronary heart disease 170
- Hypertension 174
- Asthma and bronchitis 176
- Viral rhinitis and sinusitis 179
- Tonsillitis 181
- Diarrhoea 182
- Constipation 184
- Peptic ulcer 186
- Hepatitis 188
- Obesity 191
- Diabetes 194
- Arthritis 197
- Spondylitis 200
- Herniated disc (slipped disc) 201
- Piles (haemorrhoids) 204
- Hernia 205
- Menstrual abnormalities 208
- Eye problems 211
- Stress 216
- Anxiety disorder 218
- Drug addication 219

Reference 221

Annexure 223

SECTION I

YOGA, PREKSHA MEDITATION AND HEALTH

- What is yoga 2
- Yoga philosophy 5
- Components of yoga 9
- Preksha meditation 28
- Yoga and health 37
- Therapeutic basis of yoga 43
- Therapeutic basis of Preksha meditation 48
- Nutrition and yogic diet 53

What is Yoga?

"Yoga is a system of living with sense and science, of the realization of ultimate values and altruistic mission of life. Yoga involves a harmonious order of mind, matter and man.

Yoga is an absolute departure from basic animal tendencies.

Yoga is a state of aloofness from the artificialities of life and relationship. Yoga is the culture of tomorrow!"

— *Swami Satyanand Saraswati*

'Yoga' is derived from the Sanskrit dhatu (base) 'Yuj', which means 'to join or bind', 'to attach'. It also means 'to direct' and 'to concentrate on a particular point of thought', 'to work in full attention of mind and body'. It is a true union of 'Atma' (Soul) with almighty 'Parmatma' (God). This union also includes physical, mental, intellectual and spiritual faculties of a human being. In the words of Mahadev Desai it is the "yoking of all the powers of body, mind and soul to God". He says "this means the disciplining of the intellect, the mind, the emotions, the will, that yoga presupposes; it means a poise of the soul which enables one to look at life in all its aspects evenly."

Maharshi Patanjali has given a new dimension to the age-old orthodox yoga philosophy. He collected, coordinated and illustrated the basic principles of yoga in his classical work *Yoga Sutras.* He explained yoga as "Chitta Vritti Nirodha (चित्त वृत्ति निरोध)", which means balanced mind-brain system.

According to Upanishads, yoga is the higher state of consciousness in which the activities of mind and intellect come to a stationary state and wisdom comes to a stand-still.

As stated in *Bhagvad Gita,* yoga is the freedom from all sorrows. It has also been defined as *Yoga Karmasu Kaushalam (योगः कर्मसु कौशलम्)* (*Gita* 2/50), which means yoga is a skill that does not become the reason of 'bandh' (the act of fastening to the worldly affairs). One should act without any preoccupied notions and desires. By another definition, as narrated in *Bhagvad Gita,* yoga has been described as *Samatvam Yoga Uchchyate (समत्वं योग उच्यते),* which means to act without greed for result and to remain unmoved after both success and failure is yoga. In *Bhagvad Gita,* Lord Shri Krishna explains to Arjuna that deliverance from contact with pain and sorrow is called yoga. It is mentioned that when mind, wisdom and self are well under control, freedom from desires prevails, only then one can understand the real meaning of eternal joy and that will be the condition beyond explanation. In such a condition the person abides in the real feeling and does not move even a bit. He will be free from the greatest state of agonies and sorrow. This is the real yoga.

Swami Sivananda has explained that "Yoga is integration and harmony between thoughts, words and deeds, or integration between head, heart and hands." Swami Satyanand Saraswati,* while describing yoga, has said that "from the harmony of the mental and physical aspects of man (including of course the pranic or bioplasmic body and our emotional nature) are derived other positive virtues as by-products. From these arise many other definitions of yoga. The following are a selection taken from the classical yoga text, *Bhagavad Gita*:

Yoga is equanimity in success and failure (2/48)

Yoga is skill and efficiency in action (2/50)

Yoga is supreme success of life (4/3)

Yoga is the giver of untold happiness (5/2)

Yoga is serenity (6/3)

Yoga is the destroyer of pain (6/17)"

Yoga may also by defined as the science of consciousness, the science of creativity, the science of personality development, the science of self, and the science of body and mind. Actually its meaning, definition and explanation may differ from person to person in view of varied nature of an individual's feelings and experiences. But one thing is perfectly clear that yoga is always concerned with three integrated components of self — body, mind and consciousness. It is an augmentation of facts and life knowledge, gained from experience concerning the fundamental importance of a constant state of balance.

Yoga Philosophy

Although yoga has innumerable facets, its fundamental teachings are based on philosophical and spiritual principles. Its development has taken place gradually in many phases of time, beginning from the previous knowledge stored in ancient *Upanishads, Bhagavad Gita* and the basics elaborated by Patanjali in his monumental work *Patanjali Sutras.* It has travelled and got enriched through the wisdom and thoughts of several Hindu, Jain, Buddhist and Sufi philosophical thinkers, as well as of the modern sages and saints like Swami Vivekananda, Sri Aurobindo, Pandit Sampurnananda and Mahatma Gandhi. Several scientific studies have been carried out on yoga in association with modern basic and medical sciences. Even after continuously changing scenario, the basic spiritual principles of yoga are still valid and acceptable to one and all.

Yoga Darshan and *Sankhya Darshan* are so much vividly descriptive that most of the principles (sutras) revealed there are very much valid even today. There are however certain basic differences, for example, Sankhya is sceptic whereas yoga is theistic, because it accepts the existence of almighty God (Ishwara). According to Sankhya metaphysical knowledge is the only path to salvation, whereas according to yoga it may be achieved by precious techniques of meditation. Patanjali's effort was directed especially to coordinate the philosophical material, taken from Sankhya, around technical formula for concentration, meditation and ecstasy. In fact Patanjali converted the mystical thoughts of yoga into a systematic system of philosophy, by giving it proper shape of technique, which is under reach of a human being, if tried honestly.

Both Sankhya and Yoga agree that the world is *real*;

and if it *exists* and *endures*, it is because of the *ignorance* of spirit; the innumerable forms of the cosmos as well as their processes of manifestation and development exist only in the measure to which the Self *(purusha)* is ignorant of itself, and by reason of this metaphysical ignorance, suffers and is enslaved. At the precise moment when the last self shall have found its freedom, the creation in its totality will be reabsorbed into the primordial substance.

It is here in this fundamental affirmation that the cosmos exists and endures because of man's lack of knowledge, that we can find the reason for the Indian depreciation of life and the cosmos — a depreciation that none of the great constructions of post - Vedic Indian thought attempted to hide. From the time of Upanishads, Indians denounced the world as it is and treated life as it reveals itself to the eyes of a sage — ephemperal, painful, illusory. Such a conception leads neither to nihilism nor to pessimism. *This* world is rejected, *this* life is depreciated, because it is known that *something else* exists, beyond becoming, beyond temporality, beyond suffering.

In religious terms it could be said that India rejects the *profane* cosmos and *profane* life, because it thirsts for a *sacred* world and a *sacred* mode of being. Again and again Indian texts repeat that the cause of soul's 'enslavement' and consequently the source of its endless sufferings lie in *man's solidarity with cosmos,* in his participation, active and passive, direct and indirect, in nature.

Pain Exists

Dukhmeva Sarva Vivekinah (दुःखमेव सर्व विवेकिनः), recalls Patanjali in his *Yoga Sutras.* Human being himself, with all his experiences, undergoes suffering. Aniruddha in "Commentary on Sankhya Sutras" has stated that "The body is pain, because it is the place of pain; the sense, objects and perceptions are suffering, because they lead to suffering; pressure itself is suffering, because it is followed by suffering." Basic principle of Sankhya is man's desire to escape from the pains of celestial misery, terrestrial misery and inner or organic misery.

Emancipation from sufferings remains the goal of all schools of Indian philosophies and mysticisms. This may be achieved by either means and ways. It may be obtained directly through knowledge (as directed by teachings of Vedanta and Sankhya) or by means of the techniques mentioned in Yoga Sutras and Buddhist scriptures. One fact remains very clear that a knowledge has no value if it does not seek salvation of man. (M. Eliade in *Yoga — Immortality and Freedom).*

"In Indian philosophy metaphysical awareness always contains soteriological aim, and only metaphysical knowledge — the knowledge of ultimate realities — is valued and sought, for it alone procures liberation" . (M. Eliade in *Yoga — Immortality and Freedom).* It is only the knowledge that enables a man to be 'awakened' by casting off the illusions of this world of phenomena. By knowledge is meant the practice of withdrawal, whose effect will be to make him find his own centre, to make him coincide with his *true spirit* (Purusha — atman). Knowledge is transformed into a kind of meditation, and metaphysics becomes soteriology. In India not even 'logic' is without a soteriological function in its beginning.

The importance that all these Indian metaphysical and ascetic techniques and contemplating methods that constitute yoga accord to 'knowledge' is easily explained if we take into consideration the causes of human sufferings. The wretchedness of human life is not owing to a divine punishment or to any specific sin, but due to ignorance. It however does not include every and all kinds of ignorance but only the ignorance of true nature of *spirit*, the ignorance that makes us attribute 'qualities' and predicates to the eternal and autonomous principle. Hence naturally it should be the metaphysical knowledge for leading us to the threshold of illumination, that is to the true *'self'*. And it is this knowledge of one's *self*, in its ascetic and spiritual sense, that is being pursued by a majority of Indian speculative schools; the school of yoga being one of the most effective among them.

For yoga the problem is clearly defined. Since sufferings have their origin in ignorance of *spirit* (on confusing spirit with psychomental state), emancipation can be obtained only if this confusion is abolished. For that yoga (a state of asceticism) and techniques of meditation are indispensable to obtain liberation. In yoga philosophy it is pointed out that human sufferings are rooted in illusion, for man believes that his psychomental life — activity of the senses, feelings, thoughts and volitions — is identical with *spirit*, with the *self*. In such a way he mixes two autonomous but opposite realities, between which there is no real connection but only an illusory relation. Psychomental experience does not belong to spirit, it belongs to nature whereas states of consciousness are refined products of the same substance, that is at the base of the physical world and world of life. Between psychic states and inanimate objects or living beings there are only differences of degree. But between psychic states and *spirit* there is a difference of an ontological order; they belong to two different modes of being. *'Liberation'* occurs when one has understood this truth, and when the *spirit* regains its original freedom.

———:::::::: ———

Components of Yoga

Yoga has been referred to as the age-old and regarded as the continuous, uninterrupted tradition of knowledge for several thousand years. It has been established on innumerable theories, concepts, techniques, practices and rules, which were hypothesised in various regions over many a millennium. Fundamentals of yoga are well defined in the *Kathopanishad, Bhagvad Gita* and *Yoga Sutras.* These fundamental principles of yoga, both in theory and practice, are known as *Classical Yoga* or *Ashtanga Yoga* in Indian tradition. The Astanga Yoga is comprised of eight constituents or eight limbs, which are very well defined in the Patanjali's *Yoga Sutras.* They can be classified under the following three heads:

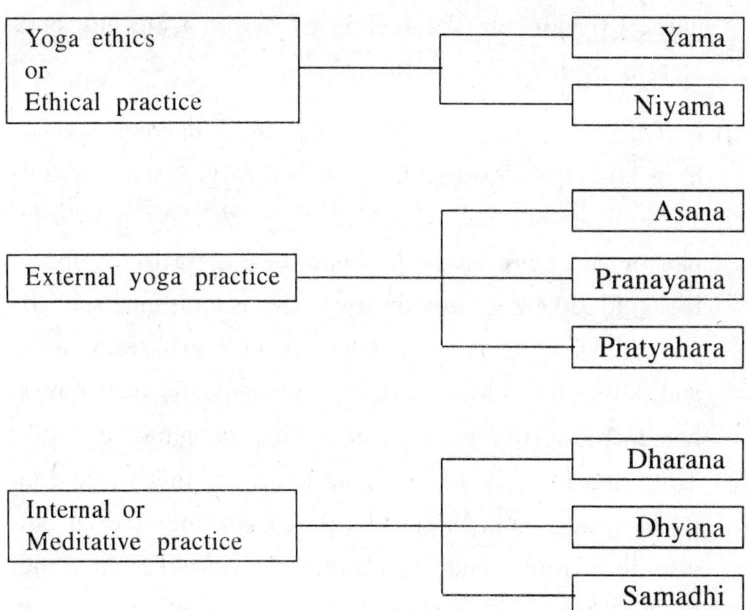

Yama

It is the first step, which includes five abstentions, namely:

- non-violence (ahimsa)
- truthfulness (satya)
- honesty (asteya)
- sexual continence (brahmacharya)
- non-acquisitiveness (aparigraha)

Ahimsa: It is universal moral commandment and is ethical preparation for a student of yoga. Not to harm any living being by any means is the basic principle of non-violence. This creates an atmosphere of universal love and brotherhood and makes the one's mind pure. To reprobate the feeling of hatred from any one is also a part of non-violence.

Satya: Truth is universal and is the only uncontroversial basis for the development of self. Mahatma Gandhi said, "Truth is God and God is Truth". As a natural phenomenon, fire burns the impurities, thereafter refining the gold; likewise fire of truth cleans our innerself. If one thinks of truth, if tongue speaks about truth only, and if one acts based on truth, automatically one moves one step ahead towards union with the almigthy God. Truth and love are the ultimate reality of this world and a yogi must adopt these realities in not only speech but also in routine conduct. Untruthfulness, either in mind or in action, leads a yogi away from his mission.

Asteya : To desist the desire of using other's belongings, whether money, thought or materials, for own benefit, is Asteya. This act of non-stealing includes not only taking what is other's without prior permission, but also using it for different purposes or using beyond the permitted time period. This also includes misappropriation, misconduct, misuse, mismanagement and breach of trust. Asteya not only gives mental peace and self-purification to an individual, but also reduces several social tensions and evils. One should reduce one's needs to the minimum, to achieve the ability to ward off great temptations.

Brahmacharya : To live the life of celibacy, to develop self-restraint and to perform religious acts are the basic principles of brahmacharya. It does not only mean to preserve semen and remain celibate. To remain strictly away from sexual activities in deed or thought is the basic principle of several abstinence components of brahmacharya. The concept of brahmacharya is not one of negation, forced austerity and prohibition. To lay stress on continence of the body, speech and mind is the real brahmacharya, as stated by Maharshi Patanjali. It has little to do with a person's marital status and living a common man's household life. It is open for all. It is not at all necessary for one's salvation to stay unmarried, because one can perform marital duties solely for the creation of progeny but not for sexual pleasures and thus still remain a brahmachari.

Aparigraha : To remain free from hoarding is Aparigraha. A yogi should keep his requirements to the minimum as he does not really need many things at a particular point of time; hence he should not hoard or collect the things. The collection of things, for future needs, shows the lack of faith in God and in himself, because he (the God) who is looking after whole creations (shristi) will fulfil and meet our requirements timely. By observing the habit of aparigraha, one makes one's life very simple, where there is no fear or lack of trust. The life of a common man is full of miseries, disturbances, agonies and frustrations, which keep his mind always in a state of imbalance and perturbation. The basic reasons for such a condition are his failure to fulfil his desires or the fear to lose something which he has hoarded for his future or for his luxury. The observance of aparigraha enables a person to remain satisfied with whatever he has and whatever happens to him. He achieves peace, which takes him beyond the realms of illusion and misery. His mind is always calm and cool, unperturbed and in a state of equilibrium.

Niyama

These are the rules (code) of conduct that apply to individual disciplines. The five niyamas discribed by Maharshi Patanjali are:

- Shauch (purity)
- Santosh (contentment)
- Tapas (austerity)
- Svadhyaya (self-study)
- Ishwara pranidhan (dedication to the God)

Shauch : For our well-being, purity of physical body is essential. At the same time cleansing of the mind of its disturbing emotions like hatred, passion, anger, lust, greed, delusion and prides, is equally important. Also the cleansing of our intellect of impure and unhealthy thoughts is equally important. The toxins and impurities of body are removed by pranayam and asanas. They not only clean the body but also tone the entire body along with its rejuvenation. The impurities of mind may be washed off by adopting devotion (bhakti), whereas the impurities of intellect are removed or burned off in the fire of self study (svadhyaya). Purification or cleansing of the physical body, mind and intellect brings the sate of benevolence (saumanasya), which banishes mental pain, dejection, sorrow and despair, and gives satisfaction with joy. In this condition the person is able to concentrate one's mind to obtain victory over one's own senses. Thereafter he enters the sacred temple of his own body and sees his real self in the mirror of his mind.

Food is the basic necessity of body. To keep the body and mind healthy, right kind of food is necessary. One should be very careful how his food is procured, how it is prepared and in what way it has been consumed? For a yogi, vegetarian diet is essential in order to attain concentration and spiritual evolution. Food is to be taken to promote health, to get energy and strength, and for the purpose of self-rejuvenation only. Hence the food should be simple, nourishing, juicy, soothing and with all necessary nutrients like carbohydrate, protein, vitamins, minerals and roughages. Sour, bitter, salty, pungent, burning, heavy and unclean food should necessarily be avoided. Besides food, our habitat is equally important for spiritual practices and healing purposes. It should be free from insects and noise pollution, airy, dry and clean.

Santosh: Santosh or contentment has to be developed. When a person is greedy for something or other, his mind cannot concentrate. One should feel happy in whatever condition one is living and whatever wealth one has (or does not have). He should be contented with what he has, and should be grateful to the God for his grace. Cast, creed and wealth are the fundamental factors for dissatisfaction among the people, and that leads to conscious or unconscious conflicts. In such conditions mind cannot concentrate or it cannot become single-minded (ekagra) and as a result it is robbed of its peace, which is not the way of tranquility, truth and joy, in whose absence no success, of whatever kind, can be achieved.

Tapas: Efforts and practice of character building may be termed tapas. It means to burn, shine, consume, blaze or destroy all kinds of pain with the help of inner self-control energy. It is a process of burning the desires that stands in the way of achieving the ultimate goal of life. It involves self-purification, self-discipline and austerity, and is a conscious effort to achieve the ultimate union with the divine. Tapas is of three kinds, that is it may be related to body (kayika), to speech (vachika) or to mind (mansika). Brahmaharya (continence) and ahimsa (non-violence) are the tapas of body. Using such words that do not offend others, reciting the glory of Almighty God, always speaking truth without thinking of its consequences are the tapas of speech. To keep tranquil and balanced in both joy and sorrow and always have self control are the tapas of mind. To work without selfish motive or hope of reward is the fundamental principle of tapas. Tapas helps in developing strong body, mind and character, which yield courage, wisdom, integrity and simplicity with straight- forwardness.

Svadhyaya: This means self-study or education. Education is a process that brings out the best; which is within ourselves. Thus the educating the self is svadhyaya. In the practice of svadhyaya the person concerned is the speaker as well as the listener. It is not a practice of class room lecture where the lecturer speaks before the audience of students who follow the instructions.

In svadhyaya people speak and listen themselves. Their mind and heart are full of love and respect, and the noble thoughts arising from this practice are taken into blood stream to make them a part of life and being. Svadhyaya changes the outlook of life. The person starts believing that all creations are divine and life is meant for adoration and not for enjoyment only. He feels that there is a part of divinity with himself and that source of energy which is engraved in him is given by God, which flows in others too.

Acharya Vinoba Bhave said that svadhyaya is the study of ourself, which is the basis or root of all other subjects, upon which the others rest, but which itself does not rest upon anything.

To lead a spiritual, healthy, peaceful and happy life, it is necessary to develop the habit of reading healthy and divine literature. It will bring to an end ignorance and misbeliefs. This habit enables the person to understand the nature of his soul and to establish the link with divine.

Ishvara pranidhana: Dedicating one's all will, wish and actions to the God is Ishvara pranidhana. He who has faith in God, who knows that all creations belong to the God, will not face any dilemma, will not be puffed up with pride or drunk with power and will bow his head only in worship. Our senses are gratified with greed and attachment, and any hindrance in this process leads to sorrow. They may be curbed with the help of knowledge and forbearance in full conscious state only. Conscious state is directly governed by mind, and to control mind is very difficult. This needs extra resources, which can be obtained from the God. For that one has to take the shelter of God with full honesty and dedication. It is at this stage that devotion (bhakti) begins. In bhakti the mind, intellect, will and wish are made subservient humbly to God with the pray that 'I' am nothing and that the Almighty will take care of me. This is feeling of 'I' and 'mine' and appearance of true love and devotion which leads the individual's soul to a full growth. When the mind is filled with the thoughts of personal gratification, there is always danger of the senses dragging the mind after the objects of desire. But when the mind is emptied of desire of personal gratification, it may easily acquire and filled with thought of God. This way of bhakti will enable the person to proceed in right direction of knowledge and conduct, because the name of God is like the sun dispelling the darkness. When our life-moon will face the sun, it will be glowing like a full moon.

Asana (Art of Postures)

In Patanjali's ashtanga yoga, after yama and niyama, the third limb is asana or posture. Asanas are well described in *Hathyoga Pradipika,* where it has been placed first in the sequence of yoga practice. "The posture in which one can sit for indefinite period comfortably is called asana", as described in *Mandal Brahmanopanishad*. Patanjali says "Sthir Sukhasanam" (स्थिर सुखमासनम), which means the posture in which we can sit comfortably and steadily is called asana. Asana brings real steadiness, health and easiness to all body parts, which ultimately bring mental equipoise and peace. They are altogether different from gymnastic exercises. One does not need any infrastructure facility or equipment to perform asana, as in case of games or gymnastic exercises. It can be performed alone and anywhere without any specific preparation. What is needed is only a small blanket, a clean and airy space and self-confidence. By practising the asanas one can develop physical health, endurance, vitality, and can achieve longevity due to perfect health.

Asanas are classified in three categories:

- Meditative asanas
- Asanas providing mental tranquility
- Asanas providing physical strength

Asanas falling in the first category are practised before meditation. They are most suitable postures for doing meditation session. The second group of asanas provide total mental peace and tranquility and prevents fickleness of mind. The third group of asanas is practised to get physical strength and body power. Asanas have been evolved over the centuries, so as to exercise every muscle, nerve and gland in the body. They help in securing a fine physique, which is strong and elastic without being muscle bound and they keep the body free from disease. They also reduce fatigue and soothe the nerves. But their real importance lies in the way they train and discipline the mind.

Every asana consists of three stages, that is coming into the prescribed pose, holding it or keeping stationary, and then coming out of it. They should be performed slowly, steadily and with patience. One should try to keep still while maintaining the pose and breathe slowly and deeply, concentrating one's mind on breath only. Once the ability to relax in a particular pose is achieved, one can adjust his position to achieve a greater stretch. Asanas are to be used for the systematic use of different muscles to get balanced coordination of physical, mental and visceral activities. According to recent scientific studies, in addition to provideing comfortable postures for concentration *(Dhyan)* and meditation *(Samadhi)*, steady body poses and body's physical development, the asanas lead to various useful physiological, biochemical and mental changes in the body. These changes include loss in body weight, decreased respiratory rate, increased vital capacity of lungs, increased chest expansion, decreased blood glucose level, decreased blood cholesterol level, increased blood protein level, improved functions of endocrine glands, and improved mental processes, like intelligence quotient (IQ), mental quotient (MQ), work efficiency, decreased mental fatigue and anxiety etc. Several other significant neurophysiological and neurohumoral changes have been reported to take place following the practice of asanas. A prefect balance between physical goodness and mental consciousness leads to good health, and a person gets health by performing asanas. In fact health is not a commodity that can be purchased by money power. It has to be achieved by self-effort and that too by sincere and systematic hard work and practice. Asanas are a means for that. They not only help a practitioner getting freedom from physical disabilities and mental distractions, but also achieve a complete equilibrium of body, mind and sprit.

Pranayama (Science of Breath)

Pranayama is the process of yogic breath or science of breath. As stated in *Yoga Sutras*, *'tasmin sati shwas prashwas yorgati vichchhedah pranayamah'* (*तस्मिन् सति श्वास प्रश्वास योर्गति विच्छेदः प्राणायामः*), that is pranayama is related with Prana, which means breath, respiration, life, vitality, wind, energy or strength. The suffix 'Ayam' means length, expansion, stretching or restraint. Pranayama thus means the extension of breath along with its control. Every breath has three components: (1) inhalation or inspiration, which is termed *Puraka* (to fill), (2) retention or holding the breath, a state where the inspired air is held in the lungs, termed *Kumbhaka,* and (3) exhalation or expiration, which is called *Rechaka* (to empty), in which the air filled in lungs is to be released quietly. There are two states of Kumbhaka, Abhyantar Kumbhaka and Bahya Kumbhaka. In the Abhyantar Kumbhaka the seeker (Sadhak) witholds the breath while he is in the stage of Puraka, and in Bahya Kumbhaka he witholds the breath in the stage of Rechaka.

In pranayama there is a measured timing ratio for the three stages and the ratio should be carefully observed.

In yogic breathing, inhalation (Puraka) consists of muscular action. The movement has two parts working together. In the first part the thoracic cage expands to make room for lungs to inflate. In the second part the dome-shaped diaphragm flattens out and descends, swelling out the abdomen and, incidentally, massaging beneficially the abdominal viscera. Now one should breathe deeply, pour air into the lungs, but the point at which the inflation and expansion ends should be just before the point at which discomfort intrudes. If one sits easily, with the back straight and in the level of head, the respiratory muscles will be free to expand and recoil in comfortable pranayama.

Holding the breath is a conscious act that checks the mechanism, whereby our respiration is automatically regulated. With conscious suspension of breath (Kumbhaka) we just switch from 'automatic' to 'manual', as it were. This requires some practice for smoothness and ease. This means refraining from forcing, and making comfort the criterion. When Kumbhaka follows filling of the lungs, the thoracic umbrella must stay open, diaphragm down and the abdomen out during the immobile breathing pause. One has to inhibit the initial tendency of the ribs and diaphragm to recoil during the full pause, and to expand and rise respectively during the empty pause. However after some weeks of training, inhibition becomes effortless as long as Kumbhaka is not prolonged to a point of strain. During Kumbhaka with full lung or empty lung, one should resist the temptation to let a little air through the nostrils or mouth to keep the suspension going comfortably. The abdomen should not change the tone by contracting or relaxing. Yogic breath suspension (Kumbhaka) achieves both physiological and psychological benefits. The pause gives more time for gaseous exchange (O_2 : CO_2) across the blood capillaries. In addition, it allows better mixing of fresh air with the stale residual air in the air sacs of the lungs. Holding of breath, during the period lungs are filled, has a cleansing and purifying effect on the residual air.

In pranayama, comprehensive time is allocated to empty the lungs as to fill them. Carbon dioxide — the waste product that all the cells of the body exchange for fresh oxygen every three minutes — is expelled from the body with the outgoing breath. Some residual air remains, as mentioned earlier. The more complete and efficient the exhalation, the more efficient the purification, and the greater the lung expansion and inflow of fresh air and oxygen on the following inspiration.

Pratyahara (Sensual Control)

If a man has firm and rhythmic control on his senses, he may be free from several agonies caused by them. This is known as Pratyahara, where the senses, which are basic source of all sensual tyrannies, are brought well under control. This is the fifth stage of yoga. To find a way to defeat the deadly spell of sensual objects, a man needs the shadow of Bhakti in which he recalls to his mind the Almighty creator of all such objects. In fact man's mind is at the central point, around which all pleasure or pain, bondage or liberation, happiness or sorrow are revolving continuously. There is bondage, pain, sorrow if one's mind indulges, grieves over any specific subject matter; and at the same time there is pleasure, liberation and happiness if mind is free from all desires and fears. The purpose of life should be to acquire the 'good' instead of 'pleasant'; but the common man goes for pleasant, losing the sacred element of the precious life. To achieve the good and sacred is the ultimate aim of Pratyahara. By practicing Pratyahara a person feels joy and satisfaction, because he knows how to stop and where to go, what to accept and what to reject. He understands that what is bitter like a poison today will become sweet tomorrow.

A man observing the principles of yoga knows that the path of sensual satisfaction and desire fulfilment goes straight to destruction, whereas to tread the path of yoga is like walking on the sharp edge of a razor. It is a narrow and difficult path to tread, and there are few who follow it, although it is the only path of salvation.

By obseving Pratyahara a person experiences the fulness of creation or of the creator, his thirst for the objects of senses vanishes, and he looks at them everafter with dispassion. He remains stable in all conditions of pain or pleasure, virtue a vice, honour or dishonour. He remains in the state of equanimity, experiencing the fullness of universal soul; and such a condition of his attitude and behaviour leads him to the path of perfection.

Dharna (Concentration)

It is the sixth stage of classical Patanjali Yoga. Dharna is the concentration on a single point, or total attention on what is to be done at a particular moment, the mind remaining unmoved and unruffled. It stimulates the inner awareness to integrate the ever-flowing intelligence and to release all tensions. In fact without concentration nothing can be achieved. Without concentration on divinity, which shapes and control the universe, one cannot unlock the divinity within oneself or become a universal man.

The mind should be the willing servant of the self. But it is only a very rare man or woman who possesses sufficient natural self-discipline for achieving this. It is usual for most of us that mind is either a helpless slave or tyrannical master. Without adequate orientation, we are all time affected with worldly abuses. Some of us let ourselves be buffeted by emotional storms or are forever being distracted by external stimuli, with the result that single - minded pursuit of what is truly important to us is all but impossible. Others tend to veer to the other extreme; in an effort to set up defenses against external or emotional distraction, we become creatures of the mind exclusively, denying natural impulses. Thus in one way or other our very efforts at self-discipline defeat us, consuming energy that could more conveniently be put to constructive and creative use. These basic failures of human nature are as old as human nature itself. The yogis, wisely aware of them, long ago devised a method for dealing with the problem, and this is the basis of the practice of *Dharna*.

In the process of concentration one must concentrate on 'something' since obviously there can be no such thing as concentration in a mental vacuum. One should focus one's attention on some image or object while determinedly shutting out everything else. Thereafter with one's mind made to dwell closely and steadily on that object or image alone, one can ultimately achieve perfection. It goes without saying that to concentrate properly one must keep serene, which means emptying the mind of irritation, worry and distraction, not permitting any of these emotions to take hold of our mind and interfere with our desired activity or goal. This too becomes a matter of practice. At first as one tries to concentrate on the object of one's choice, one will find the immediate preconceptions of daily life crowding the mental faculty and hammering for admittance. The way to deal with them is deliberately to shut them out. One should learn to watch one's thoughts dispassionately and objectively as though one may be an interested spectator, but should not permit oneself to identify with them. Then, when they begin to wander, one should shepherd them back where they wanted to be. Dull and unispired as this will seem at first — for day-dreaming and wool-gathering are a more attractive pastime than concentrating on, say the flame of a candle — the practice will soon yield rewards. It will be surprising how quickly a little mechanical exercise will enable the person to discipline his mind that when he is called on to focus on something important, something vital, it will no longer be tempted to wander at all.

Dhyana (Meditation)

Meditation is the practice by which there is constant observation of the mind. It means focusing the mind on one point, stilling the mind, in order to perceive the self. By stopping the waves of thoughts one comes to understand his true nature and discover the wisdom and tranquility that lie within. It is the seventh step of Patanjali Yoga. As focusing the rays of the sun with a magnifying glass makes them hot enough to burn an object, similarly focusing the scattered rays of thoughts makes the mind penetrating and powerful. With the continued practice of meditation one can discover a greater sense of purpose and strength of will and one's thinking becomes clearer and more concentrated, affecting the person and all his or her actions. Swami Vishnu Devanand has written, "Meditation does not come easily. A beautiful tree grows slowly. One must wait for the blossom, the ripening of the fruit and the ultimate taste. The blossom of meditation is an expressible peace that permeates the entire being. Its fruit............. is undescribable".

Using concentration as a tool, the next and final step towards true self-mastery is meditation. Yoga teaches that through meditation the individual learns to be truly and fully conscious of himself as a unit separate and distinct from all other manifestations of life, not merely in the highly personal, individualistic western sense (which all too often leads to egocentricity and uneasy self-absorption), but in a detached way that makes him immune to superficial influences. The common man, subjected daily to competitive pressures, influenced by fears and insecurities of others, easily becomes prey to anxiety or even panic while trying to live up to impossible standards artificially set up by his social milieu. But those who wisely take time to find out 'who they are', quickly lose the need to play a life-long game of "follow the leader". They learn to differentiate between what is right for them and what is not, what they really want out of life and what they have been made to believe they want. They learn to be true to themselves and through this awareness are liberated from conformity.

It is a fact that a person himself can change his mental attitude once he learns to face and stay with his problems long enough to sort out the confusions. First, he must discover what is the real 'he' in the clutter of superimposed images. Next he must decide, just as he would with an analyst's help, which of his problems he is able to do something about, and which he must learn to live with in the light of objective reality. Once he has achieved such self-knowledge, he will feel he has stopped beating his head against the wall. An inner sense of serenity will replace senseless turmoil. Meditation is less stringent than concentration. In meditation, instead of staying sternly with one point, a person is free to let the thoughts flow into his mind, provided they are germane to the main subject. Of course, in order to keep from drifting into aimless time-wasting day-dreaming or even free association of ideas, the yogi does start out, as in concentration, by deliberately focusing his mind on something specific — often a part of his body. To learn to control one's own thinking and emotions at the source, to subdue restlessness, calm the nerves and literally *will himself* to bring about what is best in him, to shut himself off from worry and all negative attitudes — these are the realistic goals of meditation which one may set up for oneself.

Two main types of meditation are described in yoga literature; they are:

- Concrete or Saguna Meditation
- Abstract or Nirguna Meditation

In Saguna meditation one tries to focus on a concrete object on which the mind can easily dwell — on an image or visual symbol, perhaps, or a mantra which brings him to unity. In Nirguna meditation, the point of focus is an abstract idea, such as the 'Absolute', a concept that is indescribable in words. Saguna meditation is dualistic — the meditator considers himself separate from the object of meditation, whereas in Nirguna meditation the meditator perceives himself as one of the objects. Regardless of whether one practices Saguna or Nirguna meditation, the end is ultimately the same — transcendence of the Gunas. As Swami Vishnu Devanand says in his teachings, "The purpose of the life is to fix the mind on the Absolute."

Thus the self knowledge brought about by systematic meditation will first become the basis for greater self-reliance and self-confidence and later will help improve every human equation of which he is a part. Through meditation one will gain a sense of perspective that will enable him to view the world around him objectively, to accept hard facts, gauge the good and the bad at their correct value and so never allow himself to be weighed down with a sense of impotence or defeat. Similarly, there will be no room in his heart for envy, jealousy, resentment or hatred, since all these emotions stem from weakness, insecurity and fear, and they are the root cause of all physical and psychosomatic disorders. Instead one will experience fresh inner strength, which will be his balance-wheel for the rest of his life and will provide corrective measures for every bodily as well mental irregularities too.

Samadhi

Samadhi is the peak of yogi's quest. At the height of meditation his body and bodily senses are at rest, as if he is in the state of sleep, although his mental faculties are fully alert, as if he has attained super consciousness state. In fact in the state of Samadhi yogi loses consciousness of his body, breath, mind, intelligence and ego. He lives in infinite peace, where his wisdom and purity, combined with simplicity and humility, shine forth.

————::::::::————

Preksha Meditation

What is Preksha Meditation?

Sampikkhae appagamappaenam (Sanskrit — Samprekseta atmanamatmana) : This aphorism from the Jaina canon *Dasavealiyam* forms the basic principle of this system of meditation, propounded by His Holiness Acharya Mahaprajna, a great thinker, philosopher and saint of today. It simply means: 'See you thyself' — perceive and realize the most subtle aspects of consciousness by your conscious mind. Hence 'to see' is the fundamental principle of this meditation process. **Preksha** means to 'perceive carefully and profoundly'. The name *Preksha dhyan* (Preksha meditation) was therefore assigned to this system. It is basically not the concentration of 'thought' but is the concentration of 'perception'.

It is conceded that both thinking (conception) as well as seeing (perception) assist in ascertaining and knowing the truth; the latter is more potent than the former. In the tenets produced by Bhagvan Mahavir, 'Perceive and Know' is given more prominence than 'Think, Contemplate and Know'. This is because perception is strictly concerned with the phenomenon of the present; it is neither a memory of the past nor an imagination of the future. Whatever is happening at the moment of perception must necessarily be a reality. The process of perception, therefore, excludes a mere 'appearance'.

One commences the practice of this technique with the perception of the body. Body contains the soul. Therefore one must pierce the wall of the container to reach the content (the Soul). Again, breathing is a part of the body and the essence of life. To breathe is to live; and so breath is naturally qualified to be the first object of our perception, whereas the body itself would become the next one. Our conscious mind becomes sharpened to perceive the internal realities in due course, and then it will be able to focus itself on the minutest and the most subtle occurrences within the body. The direct perception of emotions, urges and other psychological events will then be possible. And ultimately the entire envelopes of **karmic** matter, contaminating the consciousness, could be clearly recognised. (— Acharya Mahaprajna and Muni Mahendra Kumar).

As stated above, our conscious mind is capable of two categories of functions, viz. thinking and perceiving — conception and perception. But it is incapable of being engaged in both the categories simultaneously. One either thinks or perceives at a time. Exclusive perception of a single object can thus become an efficient tool for steadying the ever wandering mind. If one concentrates in perceiving any external object, he finds his mind steadied and his train of thoughts almost halted. Similarly, when one concentrates on the perception of one's own internal phenomena such as sensations, vibrations or even thoughts, one will realize that the mind has stopped its usual wandering and is fully engaged in perception. In the system of Preksha meditation, perception always means experience devoid of the duality of like and dislike. When the experience is contaminated with pleasure and pain, like and dislike, perception loses its primary position. (— Muni Mahendra Kumar)

The purpose of the practice of Preksha meditation is to purify the mental states. Mind is constantly choked by contaminating urges, emotions and passions. This hampers the flow of wisdom. The hurdles of uncleanliness must first be removed. When the mind is cleansed, peace of mind automatically surfaces. Balance of mind, equanimity and the state of well being (physical health) are also experienced simultaneously. So its practice also has precious therapeutic value.

Components of Preksha Meditation

Preksha meditation is an uncomplicated easy-to-learn technique of meditation. It comprises the following constituents:

- **Kayotsarga** (Total relaxation)
- **Antaryatra** (Internal trip)
- **Shwas Preksha** (Perception of breathing)
- **Sharira Preksha** (Perception of body)
- **Chaitanya Kendra Preksha** (Perception of psychic)
- **Leshyadhyan** (Perception of psychic colours)
- **Bhawana** (Auto suggestion)
- **Anupreksha** (Contemplation)

Total relaxation (Kayotsarga): It literally means abandonment of the body coupled with high degree of conscious awareness. In practice it is conscious suspension of all gross movements of the body, resulting in relaxation of the skeletal muscles and drastic reduction of metabolic activities. This physcial condition helps relieves mental tension and is an essential precondition for meditation practice. It becomes therefore the first phase of Preksha meditation, and must be practised for a few minutes at the commencement of all types of exercises. Apart from this, Kayotsarga may be independently practised daily for longer period. It one learns and practises systematic relaxation everyday, he would remain relaxed, calm and unperturbed in any situation. Physically, it is more restful than sleep and is direct antidote to psychosomatic maladies resulting from tension. Spiritually, in this process the lifeless body is cast off, whereas the consciousness soars upwards, freed from and outside its material shell. Thus it is not only total relaxation, but actual perception of the self, quite apart from the material non-self, i.e. the body.

Internal trip (Antaryatra) : It follows Kayotsarga. Exertion in systematic meditational discipline needs good deal of bioelectrical and nervous energy, and its generation in the system itself is essential. Spinal cord is an integral part of Central Nervous System. Its bottom is in the vicinity of Shakti kendra, i.e. Centre of energy. In the practice of Antaryatra, the conscious mind is motivated to travel from Shakti kendra to Jnana kendra (Centre of knowledge, located at the top of head, in the vicinity of cerebral cortex en route spinal cord) repeatedly. This results in an increased upward flow of vital bioelectrical energy, which may be used for better practice of meditation.

Perception of breathing (Shwas preksha) : Breathing is essential for metabolic functioning of the body. It is linked with conscious mind. Since mind is ever restless, it is extremely difficult to steady the wandering mind directly. An efficient and easy way to control mental activity is concentrated prerception of breath — Shwas Preksha. Complete awareness of breathing and nothing else but breathing is its basis. Shallow, hasty and irregular breathing must first be regulated to a deep, slow, calm and rhythmic, state. Very slow inhalation and complete exhalation, with the help of diaphragm, is called **dirgha shwas**, deep breathing. Attention can be kept focused on a single point in the respiratory tract, e.g. nostrils, or it can travel the entire tract during inhalation as well as exhalation. Various facets of breathing, such as movement of diaphragm, rate of breathing and depth of breathing can conveniently become the object of Shwas Preksha. It may be practised in two ways, viz. dirgha shwas and samvritti shwas preksha. As mentioned above, dirgha shwas is slow and complete exhalation and deep inhalation. A practitioner of dirgha shwas would be able to perceive in advance the onslaught of rising passions, and thus will be prepared to nullify their attack by resorting to such a practice. The rising passions would then begin to subside. Thus, by blunting the sharpness of their attack, a practitioner may save himself from being the victim of the dreadful urges and emotions.

In samvritti shwas preksha, breath is exhaled through one nostril and inhaled through the other, alternating again and again. Throughout the process, the perceptive mind is closely linked with the breath, which is regulated to be rhythmic. This, in turn, helps in developing the inherent capacities of the subconscious mind such as extra-sensory perception or clairvoyance.

Perception of the body (Sharir preksha) : Sharir preksha is basically a centripetal process, in which each and every constituent cell of the body is permeated by the spiritual self, that is each of them becomes sensitive and capable of carrying out metabolic function more efficiently through improved biochemical and bioelectrical actions. A totally impartial perception of the mass of sensations within the body is 'direct perception' of the psyche and the spiritual self. On physical level it helps each cell to revitalize itself. On mental level it is a methodology for training the mind to concentrate on internal phenomena instead of wandering about externally. On spiritual level, impartial perception of ever changing biological functions of the body is a means of experiencing the substratum of consciousness through its modes and attributes.

Perception of psychic centres (Chaitanya kendra preksha): Endocrine and nervous systems are two very important control systems of body. Though endocrine system works as the seat of the impulses and emotions, the nervous system translates and puts into action the code of intangible and imperceptible forces of the psyche with the help of nerves and muscles. Integrated functions of these two systems governs the physical and mental state, behaviour and habits of an individual. A peculiar functional interlocking between these two systems has provided a basis to treat them as one integrated system, called *neuro-endocrine system.* It is this system that comprises the subconscious mind, and profoundly influences psychological behaviour and tendencies of the conscious mind. It is therefore obvious that to cleanse the psyche by removing psychological distortions we have to find means of transforming the nature of the chemical messengers, known as *hormones*, which come from endocrine system.

In the system of Preksha meditation several psychic centres (Chaitanya kendras) are described corresponding to different endocrine glands, as follows:

Endocrine glands	**Chaitanya kendras**
Pineal	Jyoti kendra
Pituitary	Darshana kendra
Thyroid	Vishuddhi kendra
Thymus	Anand kendra
Adrenal	Taijas kendra
Gonads	Swasthya kendra and Shakti kendra

Perception of these psychic centres (Chaitanya kendras) will bring the development of the endocrine glands, which can modify the synthesization of the endocrine output, which in turn will establish not only firm control of the reasoning mind over all actions but also correct the imbalanced psychosomatic and metabolic activities. The cumulative effect of developing the reasoning mind and weakening the forces of the primal drives would ultimately bring about the desirable transformation in physical health, mental state, behaviour and habits.

Perception of psychic colours (Leshya dhyan) : Leshya (colour) is the agency that transforms the imperceptible micro-vibrations of the primal drives into perceptible forces, which produces appropriate conditions in the neuroendocrine system, thus acting as a liaison between the spiritual self and the physical self of a living organism. The integrated action of the endocrine system and the nervous system produces hormones and neuro-transmitters which not only generate feelings but also command appropriate action that satisfy the need of the urge. We either progress or retrogress, depending upon whether we control and subdue our primal drives or succumb to them. The process is of subduing the forces which countermand them by conscious reasoning. It is the authority of the spiritual self that commands the reasoning mind to produce the counter vibrations. The vibrations of waves resulting from the primal drives are malevolent **'leshyas'**, whereas the counter vibrations produced by the authority of the self are benevolent **'leshyas'.**

The spiritual progress will depend upon the degree of transformation of the malevolent trinity into the benevolent one. Without actual transformation, there will be no progress. This is not merely a speculation, but the basis of a real experience. And to bring about the desired transformation, perception of psychic colours — **Leshya dhyan**, has proved to be a practical means of transformation.

Autosuggestion and contemplation (Bhawana and Anupreksha) : Preksha dhyan is a comprehensive system of meditation. Though perception and awareness are primarily used for concentration, concentration of thought, i.e. contemplation, is not excluded. Thus the system of Preksha meditation bifurcates into: (a) concentration of the perception and (b) concentration of thought, i.e. 'Preksha' and 'Anupreksha'. In the former technique of meditation, perception is primarily used for concentration, whereas in the latter the conscious mind is encouraged to concentrate on a thinking process, i.e. contemplation. Both the techniques are competent to develop practitioner's conscious reasoning and modify one's attitude and behaviour.

Whenever one concentrates on a single theme and takes a purely objective view, acuity of his cognition increases manifold. Ancient philosophers used this technique extensively for realising the truth. Modern science also uses this process to ascertain the ultimate structure of the material objects.

Exercise of auto-suggestion is based on the practical application of faith and belief. The exercise brings about the necessary change in the body chemistry, thereby weakening the forces of disease and ultimately curing it. The principle of contemplative meditation shows the way to the practitioner to sublimate and coordinate the enhanced vital energy obtained after observing earlier steps of Preksha meditation. There are various facets of eternal truth to choose from. An experienced practitioner would know which facet he should contemplate upon. Thus he would be able to maintain his equanimity and balance even under the most aggressive state.

Yoga and Health

Yoga is a complete science of health, which deals with the understanding of the adequate functioning of all systems of our body and appropriate coordination between them, along with the healthy functioning of our mind. It differs from the western medicine in the sense that this system deals basically with the disease, its diagnosis and treatment. The techniques of yoga are designed in such a way that they not only maintain but also enhance the potentiality of body parts, which yield good health, vitality, disease-free and lasting youthfulness. Regular practice of yoga not only keeps the body healthy and fit, but also prevents either of the physical, mental and emotional imbalances due to various reasons in our day-to-day life. In natural state, if all components of the body perform their functions adequately, that will be termed as state of health. In case of any disorder and abnormality every such part works to restore the health. A device that promotes such restoration phenomena may prove to be of great importance. Yoga is foremost of them.

There are three major subdivisions in the structural organisation of the body. First subdivision, known as 'infrastructural group', includes skeleton, muscular and integumentary systems; the second subdivision, known as 'control group', includes nervous and endocrine systems, and the third subdivision is termed 'maintenance group', which includes the remaining systems, viz. respiratory system, digestive system, excretory system, cardiovascular system, immune system, lymphatic system and reproductive system. In the state of health, in spite of a number of variations in their structure, all these systems work in very balanced coordination. Yoga works systematically on all these systems to keep them functioning in better balance and perfect condition.

Much of the illness and loss of vitality are the result of bodily abuses, which we undertake knowingly or unknowingly. In today's mechanised life we spend long hours without proper air, sunlight, adequate sleep, adequate relaxation and stretching various body parts, balanced diet and planned activities, which leads to unending series of troubles and ailments. Yoga can do much more to restore normal biological, biochemical and mechanical activities of body systems, even after quite unhealthy life style for years together.

Yoga philosophy has very vast dimension, and physical body is only one aspect. Mind and spirit are other equally vital aspects of complete health. Yoga always pays attention to integrate the functions of mind, body and spirit. According to ancient Indian philosophy there are five **"sheaths"** to human existence. The first and the innermost is **physical body**; the second is the **vital body**, known as **Prana**, through which vital energy flows throughout the **nadis**; the third sheath is known as **mind,** which is the seat of emotions and thoughts; fourth sheath is of perfect thought and knowledge, termed **intellect**; and the last and outermost sheath is known as **'bliss'**, which includes universal consciousness.

Different diseases and disorders originate in the imbalance in these sheaths of existence. In the first three sheaths, i.e. physical, prana and mind, ego consciousness predominates and therefore harmony in these sheaths can be easily disturbed. The fourth and fifth sheaths are parapeted by a wider, universal consciousness and cannot be permeated. When a person is truly healthy, the positive energy in the highest sheath percolates freely through the lower ones and brings total harmony and balance to all his faculties. But though the harmony of the higher sheaths is constant, the free movement of bliss can be blocked by imbalances in lower sheaths. (— Dr R. Nagrathna, Dr H. R. Nagendra and Dr R. Monro)

Yoga and Common Ailments

It has been said by the Indian yogis that 'life is the self'. In its true nature, the self is shining, perfect, spotlessly pure and without sin. But when it took on material form — a body — it acquired the sin of matter, the sin of the world. The **self,** this eternal spring of **life,** in complete equilibrium and perfect harmony, uniformly radiates the energy of life into the body. If a person's consciousness is developed equally in every direction, even if on a low level, life energy will flow uniformly into his body. The body will remain well because of equilibrium between positive and negative currents. The condition of consciousness of the individual acts as a filter, which distributes the radiated life energy into various mental and nervous centres known as **chakras**, in the class of yoga. When, for any reason, the consciouness departs from a uniform balanced development, there is a shift in the life forces, and the equilibrium ceases. However, the radiation of the supreme self with its perfect balance endeavours to smooth out the irregularities, and with tremendous strength it forces its way past the irregular distribution of energy. This levelling out of irregularities, this struggle for the re-establishment of order, is the state of disease.

Health is the natural and prerequisite condition for the body. Life force is not only dependent upon the conscious will to live a happy and healthy life, but also active as subconscious life instinct. Life force is constantly active in us. It smooths out irregularities and preserves our health; though the mankind, day after day, defiantly tramples under foot the golden rules of healthy living. The urge for self preservation has only one purpose, and there can be no disagreement about it, this urge demands life and health.

Hath yoga teaches us how to utilize, store and promote free flow of life force to the maximum extent. Whoever follows the rules of Hath yoga will never be sick and will enjoy complete health until old age. One of the most important prerequisites, however, is to get acquainted with all manifestations of life force and to learn how these can be developed and shaped; in a word, how we can put these energies to work for our consciousness.

The unilateral development of consciousness or the stagnation of the latter can also be the cause of numerous serious psychosomatic diseases and disorders. Our body and mind remain healthy when the positive current of life force manifesting itself on the material plane — in our body — is in perfect equilibrium with the negative force, the force of resistance of the body. In such a condition, there is a balance between the life force and the resistance of the body that carries it. In an individual on a low level of consciousness, the tension of life force streaming into his body is low. His control systems are adjusted to the corresponding resistance. With the expansion of consciousness, the tension of life force increases and consequently the power of the resistance of control systems must increase. If this is done step by step in complete equilibrium, the controls have time to strengthen themselves, parallel with the increasing tension of life current, and to develop corresponding resistance. If, however, the development takes place haphazardly the control becomes ill because of the lack of its own development. The aim of yoga is to make our own consciousness dependent on our will, to expand it systematically, intentionally, from one step to another, and at the same time to increase and strengthen the resistance of the circuit, which carries the constantly growing life energy.

Hath yoga exercises have a wonderful effect on the struggle against all kinds of fear. This provides the basis of physical self-control. It is well known that the body reacts to every mental impulse. Primarily this is done by nervous system and endocrine gland system, which are highly developed for the preservation of life. It has been scientifically proved that various vegetative functions depend primarily on the condition of the endocrine glands' secretion, i.e. hormonal profile of the body. If this activity is some how diminished or becomes irregular, the result is serious diseases. Thus the emotions and passions, through their destructive effect on the endocrines, are the implacable enemies of health.

In the school of yoga the endocrine glands are the locations of **chakras**. These chakras are the connecting link between mind and body. If one knows the role these chakras play in the distribution of force and storing of energy, that means he knows the kind of reaction that the maintenance of a mental condition will cause in the body by acting on those endocrine glands. In this he can get acquainted with the more intimate relationship between various mental conditions and the different organs of the body, in turn he gains control over the body and health.

The prevention and healing of disease and preservation process of health begins in the mind. And here we encounter the important role of the inter-relationship of *mind* and *body*. Therapeutic role of Hath yoga is based on this relationship and it develops, in parallel, the individual's abilities and physical health. Yoga teaches us how to keep order among the forces that animate our body and, in case we have sinned against our health through unnatural living, how we can restore our physical well being again.

———:::::::———

Therapeutic Basis of Yoga

Yoga has established its worth, since thousands of years, in elevating the status of spiritual aspects and health. But its utility in the treatment of various diseases and disorders is yet to be established. Basically, yoga is not a therapy, but for the last couple of decades, on the basis of the outcome of several scientific and medical studies, it has been emphasised that yogic exercises are quite useful in the treatment of many diseases. Also, it works as complementary and co-therapy measure in association with medicinal therapy. Yogic exercises are effective in the health recovery, diagnosis and treatment of diseases, in the patient suffering from various systemic psychosomatic disorders / diseases in three ways, as mentioned below:

- Psychotherapeutic and relaxative effect
- Physiotherapeutic and rehabilitative effect
- Cleansing effect

For therapy, appropriate yogic exercises and kriyas may be selected to influence both the body and mind of a healthy man or a patient suffering from any specific disease. Obviously the therapist or the doctor must know the physiological and biochemical effect of those exercises along with the pathological changes taking place from time to time during the state of disease or therapy. Without adequate work plan and related knowledge, such a therapeutic measure (prescribing yogic exercises) may prove harmful. It is also equally important to evaluate any possible negative effect, if at all, of those yogic exercises, in specific conditions. Only then a viable, successful and safe system of yoga therapy could be developed and established.

Three decades ago, for the first time, the world fame **Yogacharya Swami Kuvalyanand** from Lonavala, Pune (Maharashtra) and Dr Vinekar have published their results based on the studies conducted in the field of yoga therapy. Swami Kuvalyanand described the nature of health and disease based on the concepts of ancient yoga shastras, and presented few positive aspects of yoga therapy.

Prof. Ram Harsh Singh, an eminent yoga scholar and Director, Malaviya Yoga Kendra, BHU, Varanasi, has expressed the view that according to yoga and Ayurveda *microcosm* and *macrocosm,* man and his environment, are of the same nature. Human being is a unit of the whole universe (Brahmand) and it contains all those elements that constitute the universe. Microcosm and macrocosm are busy interacting and affecting each other continuously. Human being remains healthy till this interaction is in a homeostatic state. But he (man) becomes diseased at the occurrence of any imbalance in that homeostatic state and also his environment becomes polluted and damaged, which ultimately results in imbalanced human body and mind, termed disease. The correction of such imbalances in body and mind will require the correction of disturbed interaction between micro-and macrocosm. That is the basis of both Ayurveda and yoga therapy systems — Rogastu dosha vaishamyam dosha sammamrogata (रोगस्तु दोष वैषम्यं दोष साम्ममरोगता). In other words, this principle is known as **Natural Rehabilitation**.

Swami Kuvalyanand has opined that there are two main reasons of diseases in human body:

1. Deterioration in the normal process of blood circulatory and lymph circulatory process, which causes the unwanted retention of toxic substances

in the internal body tissues. Such obstruction leads to the highly increased toxicity in the body parts.

2. Imbalanced and uncoordinated neuro-muscular, neuro-endocrine and psychoneuro-immunological activities. Both these above mentioned chain of activities are complementary to each other and invariably affect each other. Whenever there is a lack of coordination between these processes, it will lead to a pathological state in the body. In such conditions only yoga therapy may not be of much use. It then essentially needs medical aid. But in addition to that, well-thought yogic exercises and yogic therapy would improve the outcome of benefit. According to **yoga shastra**, yoga therapy emphasizes the promotion of immune capacity in the body, rather than concentrating on the factors causing diseases. For this, both body and mind are being prepared for cleansing, adjustment and adaptation processes.

According to Swami Kuvalyanand, "yogic therapy provides four-fold assistance in curing our ailments —

- By developing adequate mental state
- By rehabilitating neuro-muscular, neuro-endocrine, psycho-neuro-immunological mechanisms
- By adopting healthy diet and life style
- By natural cleansing activities and by internal cleansing using 'shat kriyas'

All these activities are interdependent and complementary to each other. In fact complete benefit of these activities may be obtained when they are being applied jointly, because a living unit (body) is a unified field of body, mind and consciousness".

We find that yoga is fundamentally different from western conventional medical practice both in its approach to health care and in its modality. In conventional medical practice attention is being paid to short cut the singular factor of disease and then its correction by using specific means, whereas in yoga it is aimed to cure the illness by improving health at the level of body, mind and consciousness, and simultaneously restoring the inner harmony. Any ailment is the outcome of total imbalance in the basic organisation and coordination among earlier mentioned sheaths (koshas) of existence. The primary disrupting influence may take place at one level in the beginning but it may spread soon to other levels. Any stimuli affecting the mind soon spread to the *body* (Annamaya Kosha). In a particular profession a specific condition makes a person aggressive or mentally irritated, which simultaneously increases stress level, resulting in unusual high metabolic rate, increased muscular activity and significantly increased sympathetic response. This may lead to loss of body's stored energy and thereafter physical weakness. It is evident here that problem starts at mental level but it goes on affecting the whole body physiology. Sometimes such problems are of very serious nature and cause chronic pathological state. (— Swami Kuvalyanand)

In yoga therapy there are all useful components that take account of every aspect of the existence, i.e. body and mind together: **Shat kriyas** are effective, eliminative and purificatory measures; **asanas** relax and tone the muscles and give massage to the internal organs; **pranayama** regulates the breathing and inflow of *prana*; **meditation** brings about calm and peace of mind, pacifies the emotion and upgrades the internal spirit to heal. By this way if any negative stimuli cause imbalances, self generated positive thinking not only inhibits the spread of disruption, it also dominates in counteraction. Augmented yogic exercises, asanas, pranayama and meditational techniques, when perfomed in a planned manner with a specific purpose, prove to be much more effective.

All the components of yoga tend to give ample amount of benefits. They are not only curative elements, but also proved to be preventive devices, for all types of psycho-somatic disorders. This is the precious essence of yoga therapy. Regular practice of relevant and required yogic exercises keeps the body and mind healthy, restores natural internal balance and harmony and, in case of any disease, systematic yoga sessions of relevant techniques correct the abnormality and bring back the normal healthy state.

———— :::::::: ————

Therapeutic Basis of Preksha Meditation

Therapeutic thinking is another aspect of yoga therapy. The effect of emotions and urges on human action is stronger than that of theoretical knowledge. The effect of emotion can be subjugated by self-discipline and self-mastery. Since the obstruction to self-mastery lies deeper than conscious mind, in order to attain it one must tap the power that lies deeper in the subconscious. Fortunately, to make the effort to perform this difficult task is inherent in all people. Therapeutic thinking is a process of catharsis, which purges the psychological distortions. It is psychotherapy to cure physical, mental and emotional sickness of the individuals. It is a proper and powerful therapy to annihilate the root cause of various disorders. Once the root cause of physical diseases, mental imbalances and emotional distortions are removed, there will emerge a state of unprecedented calmness in an individual.

Application of therapeutic thinking, autosuggestion and faith healing is as ancient as mankind itself. Franz Masmer provided the link between the ancient healing techniques with modern faith healing. Ample evidence is available to prove that suggestions given to self under deep relaxation can produce striking and significant alterations in the subject's body and mental behaviour. Actually the healing power lies wholy within the person's own organisation. In the system of Preksha meditation practice of concentration of thought

(**Anupreksha**) is being performed to acquire the desirable virtues and eradication of psychological distortions by therapeutic thinking and autosuggestion. Such practice enables a practitioner to relax the mind and release suppressed emotions thereby attaining both physical and mental health.

Pathway of Preksha therapy

The mechanism of Preksha therapy is based on fundamental principle of the correction of imbalances and perversions occurring at either levels of multilayered human existence. It aims at uninterrupted self awareness. Pure stream of consciousness interacting with *micro body* (Records of informations) moves forward and energy flows in the form of *Adhyavasaya* (Primal drives). This energy flow then enters into the astral body and takes the form of electromagnetic radiation (Leshya). Streaming into *physical body* (Gross body) it affects the endocrine glands and expresses itself in the form of emotions. This further activates the nervous system, thereby generating bioelectrical impulses, and ultimately initiates various vocal and physical activities (Fig. 1).

Negative informations coming out of the inside information record room cause imbalance in energy flow and lead to dim, gloomy and dark electromagnetic radiations. They enter into physical body first at endocrine system and change the endocrine orchestra, particularly boosting lower endocrine glands, viz. adrenals and gonads. This manifests in the form of negative emotions, which compels the man

Fig. 1. (a) **Pathway of Preksha therapy**

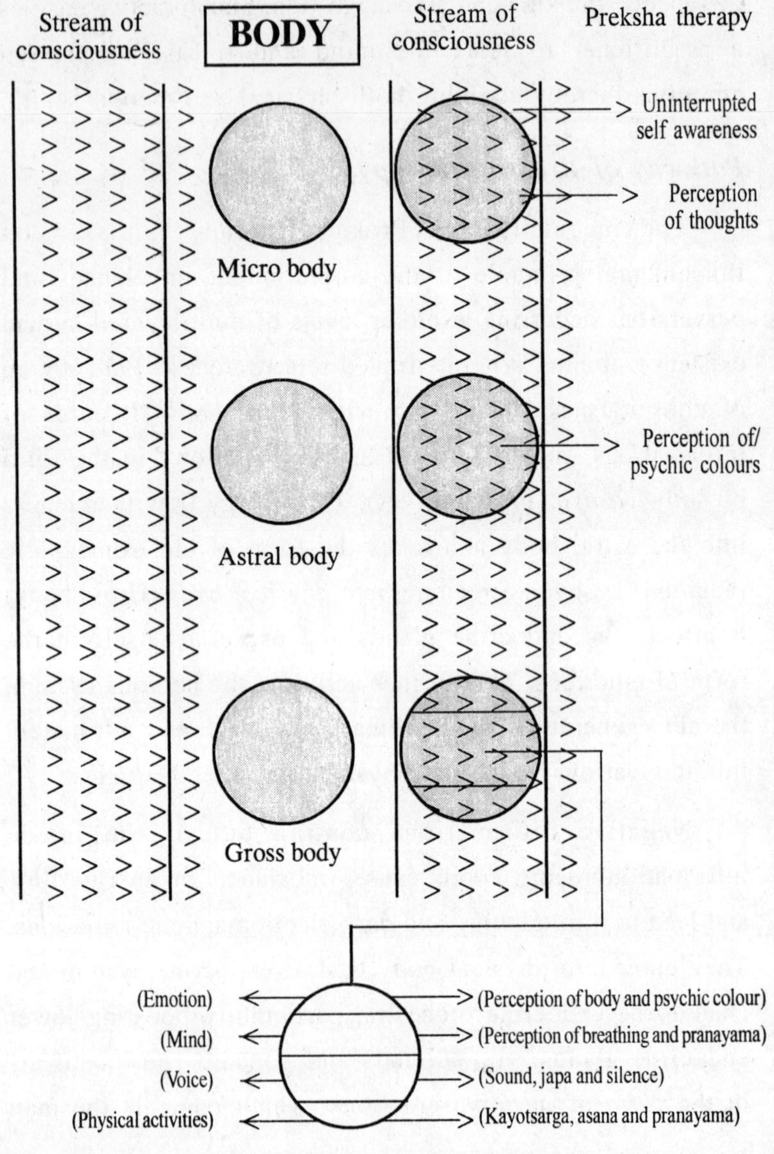

Fig. 1. (b) Pathway of Preksha therapy

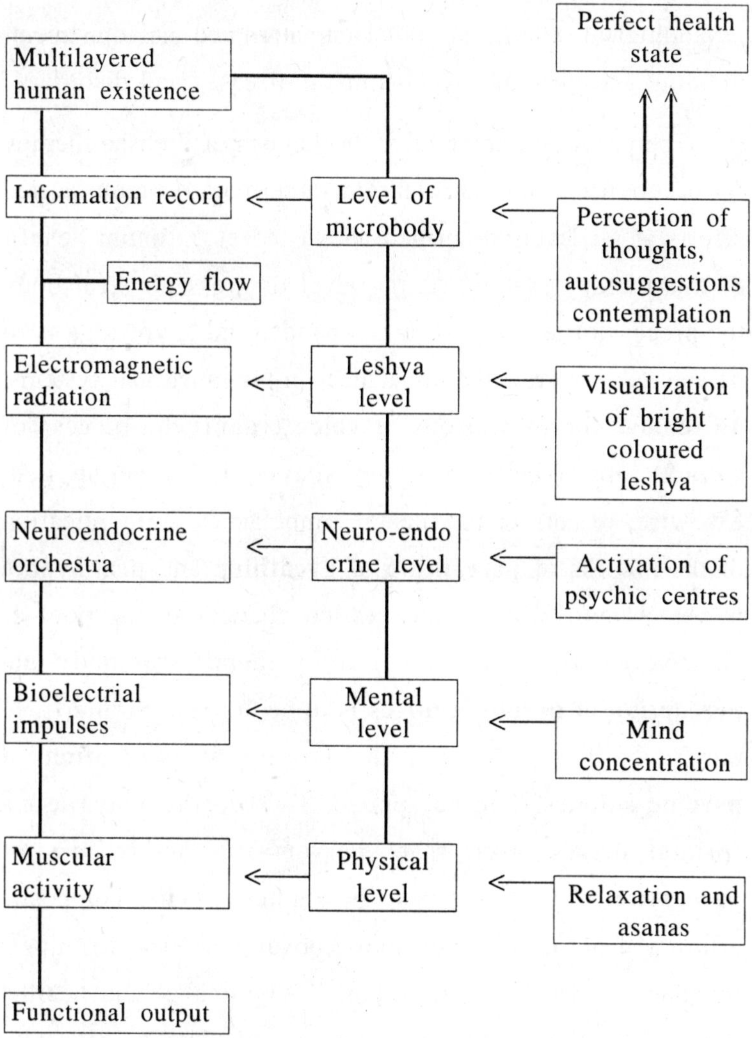

(***Source:*** **Therapentic Thinking,** by Arun Zaveri, Arham Consultants, Mumbai, INDIA).

for a variety of actions at physical and mental levels. The ultimate result is mental conflict and stress. The unresolved psychological state leads to maladaptation and maladjustment, yielding a variety of psychosomatic diseases and disorders.

The pathway of corrective mechanism of Preksha therapy for occurrence of any imbalance/disorder requires multifaceted efforts at all levels described above to get optimum benefit of this therapy system. At the level of gross physical body the process of asana, mudra and bandh, and kayotsarga is to be applied to correct the imbalances in the functional systems. To remove the perversions of **voice (vaani)** the process of **sound, japa (recitation)** and **silence** is to be applied. Likewise, to correct the mental imbalances the application of the process of **perception of breathing** and **pranayama** is prescribed. To bring the desired changes in the pool of negative emotions, the process of **perception of body** and **perception of psychic centres** is to be applied. Similarly, to purify the leshya system, the process of **perception of psychic colours** is to be applied. To keep the adhyavasaya (primal drives) free from perversion, the process of **perception of thoughts** is to be applied. Such a composite effort will not only ensure the removal of all shortcomings/ imbalances, but also bring about an optimal sound healthy state without any external invasive aid. The multilayered human existence and pathway of preksha therapy is summarised Fig. 1.

Nutrition and Yogic Diet

Diet plays a very important role in the successful practice of yoga. There is a saying, "the healthy man satisfies his hunger when he eats, the sick man satisfies his appetite." In fact "we are what we eat" — this statement is very true in more than one sense. Food is of course necessary for our physical well being, but it exerts an equal effect on our mental state. Since the outcome of mental process has direct bearing on our physical health, we cannot take it (diet) as an instrument affecting physical health only. In the recent times people are becoming more conscious about their diet and dietary habits. Modern food items like hamburgers, pizzas, jams, jellies, cola-drinks, chocolates, ice-creams, noodles etc. have gained excessive popularity due to publicity through media. It has been publicised through electronic media that such foods are much more convenient, economic, easy to procure and have so-called nutritive value too. In addition to that, canned, refined, frozen, artificially flavoured fast foods are becoming much popular among all the categories of people. Use of such foods is becoming a status symbol. It is a well-known fact that nature has provided us several nutritious edible foods in their natural form; still the people are running behind the false propaganda about so-called 'Junk-foods', without knowing about the hidden danger. It is necessary to know about the dietary habits and nurtitional requirement of our body. A brief account of nutrients and their functions, dietary patterns and digestive process is being given here.

Nutrients

Man needs a wide range of nutrients to perform various functions in the body and to lead healthy life. These nutrients include protein, fat, carbohydrate, vitamins and minerals.

These are chemical substances present in the food items. Different food items contain various nutrients in various proportions. Depending on the relative concentration of these nutrients foods are classified as protein-rich foods, carbohydrate — rich foods and fat-rich foods etc. Some foods provide only a single nutrient as in case of sugar, which is a source of only carbohydrate, whereas oils, ghee etc. provide only fats.

Carbohydrates: Carrohydrates are a class of energy yielding substances, which include starch, glucose, cane sugar, milk etc. Cereals are the main source of carbohydrates. Grain foods, roots and tubers are largely composed of starch, a complex carbohydrate. Food ingredients like simple sugars, namely cane sugar and glucose, are pure carbohydrates. Starch is a complex carbohydrate made up of glucose units. Glucose derived from starch and other sugars present in the diet is the main source of energy in the body. Carbohydrates derived from cereals form the chief source of energy in Indian diets. Starches when eaten in cooked form are completely digested in the gastrointestinal tract, and the released glucose is absorbed and metabolised in the body to yield energy.

Many other food items contain non-digestible carbohydrates like cellulose, hemicellulose, gums, pectins and lignins. These undigestible carbohydrates are designated *dietary fibre* or *unavailable carbohydrates*. These are not digested in the digestive tract and most of them are voided as such and thus contribute to the bulk of stool. Though they do not contribute to the nutritive value of foods, the presence of fibres, i.e. roughages, in the diet is necessary for the mechanism of digestion and elimination of water. The contraction of muscular walls of the digestive tract is stimulated by the fibre, thus counteracting the tendency to constipation. Lack of adequate dietary fibre in diets containing refined foods leads to constipation and intestinal cancer.

Some of the dietary fibres like gums and mucilages in our diets have been shown to lower the blood-cholesterol and blood glucose levels. Vegetables, particularly the leafy ones, fresh fruits and unrefined cereals, are comparatively rich in fibre and a generous inclusion of these helps avoid constripation.

Fats: Fat is an important component of diet and serves a number of functions in the diet. It is a concentrated source of energy and it supplies per unit weight more than twice the energy furnished by either protein or carbohydrate. It also imparts palatability to a diet and retards stomach-emptying time. Presence of fat in the diet is important for the absorption of fat-soluble vitamins like *vitamin-A* and *beta-carotene* present in the diet. Apart from these functions, some fats, particularly those derived from vegetable sources, provide what is known as *essential fatty acids*, which have vitamin-like functions in the body. Fats also form protective layers, which shield the delicate body organs from injury and allow storage of energy for future use. *Oil* and *ghee* are the main sources of fat.

In recent years there has been a revival of interest in the nutritional aspects of fats. The excessive intake of fat in diet increases the level of cholesterol in blood, which gradually leads to its being deposited under the lining of blood vessels, resulting in the condition known as *atherosclerosis,* in which the blood vessels are narrowed and hardened. The coronary arteries supplying blood to the heart are affected, leading to coronary heart disease (CHD).

In deciding the desirable level of fat in the diet, the following facts must be kept in mind:

(a) the minimum amount of fat to meet the essential fatty acid requirement

(b) the amount needed to promote absorption of fat-soluble vitamins

(c) providing palatability to food

(d) the undersirable effect of excessive intake of fat.

Proteins: Proteins are vital to any living organism. They are important constituents of tissues and cells of the body. They form the important component of muscle and other tissues and vital body fluids like blood. The proteins in the form of enzymes and hormones are concerned with a wide range of vital metabolic processes in the body. Proteins supply the body building material and make good the loss that occurs due to wear and tear. Proteins as **antibodies** help the body in defending against infection. Thus proteins are vital to the living process and carry out a wide range of functions essential for the sustenance of life and for sound health. The proteins needed by the body have to be supplied through the diet we consume. The adequacy of protein in the diet is an important measure of adequacy and quality of a diet.

Although most of the foods contain protein to varying degree, pulses, milk and milk products, oilseeds, nuts, meat, fish and eggs are the major sources of protein. In the vegetarian system of diet, pulses and milk are such an important source of protein, which is not only under reach of a common man, but also constitute most suitable food for the health of both body and mind.

1. *Biological value of proteins:* In judging the adequacy of dietary proteins to meet the human needs, not only the quantity, but the nutritional quality of the dietary proteins also matters. Proteins present in different foods vary in their nutritional quality because of differences in their **amino acid** composition. Amino acids are the building blocks of proteins. There are 22 of them in proteins, nine being designated as **essential amino acids**, since they cannot by synthesised in the body. The rest of the amino acids are called **non-essential** as they can be formed in the body by interconnections of other essential amino acids or synthesised from other simple compounds. The quality of dietary protein depends on the pattern of essential amino acids it supplies. The best quality protein is the one that provides essential amino acid pattern very close to the pattern of tissue protein. Thus biological value of a particular protein depends upon absorption and net protein utilization.

2. *Protein requirement :* Proteins are required for general maintenance, to replace the wear and tear in tissues in adults; for growth in infants and children; for foetal development in pregnancy and milk output during lactation. The relative requirements of proteins of the latter groups are higher than of adults. The actual amount of protein

to be consumed daily to meet the above-mentioned requirement will depend upon the quality of dietary protein. The higher the quality, lower the require- ment and vice-versa.

Vitamins: Vitamins are organic substances present in small amount in foods. They are required for carrying out many vital functions of body and many of them are involved in the utilization of the major nutrients like proteins, fat and carbohydrates. Although they are needed in small amount, they are essential for health and well being of the body. When these vitamins were discovered on the basis of their function, and before their chemical nature was fully elucidated, they used to be designated by affixing the letter A, B, C, D or in terms of their major functions, viz. antixerophthalmic, antineuritic, antiscorbic and antirachatic vitamins. After establishing the chemical nature of these vitamins, they are now referred to by their chemical names such as retinol, thiamine, riboflavin, ascorbic acid and cholecalciferol.

Vitamins can be broadly classified as:

(i) Water-soluble vitamins

(ii) Fat-soluble vitamins

Water-soluble vitamins are:

(a) B-complex vitamins (B_1, B_2, B_6, B_{12}, etc.)

(b) Vitamins C (ascorbic acid)

Water - soluble vitamins are not accumulated in the body, but are readily excreted, whereas fat-soluble vitamins are stored in the body. For this reason excessive intake of fat-soluble vitamins can prove toxic.

Summary chart of the important vitamins, their functions and sources is given here:

Vitamin	Prime source	Chief functions
Vit. A	Butter, whole milk egg, green leafy vegetables, red palm oil	(i) Visual process (ii) Integrity of epithelial tissues
Vit. B	Yeasts, outer layers of cereals (rice, wheat and millets), nuts, fruits, vegetables, milk, egg, meat	Antineuritic or anti beri
B-complex (B_2, B_6 etc.) (riboflavin, nicotinic acid, pantothenic acid, folic acid)	Milk and milk products; egg, green leafy vegetables, cereals, pulses, nuts	(i) Energy and protein metabolism (ii) Psychomotor development (iii)Multiplication and maturation of RBC
B_{12}	Animal foods	(i) Maturation of cells (ii) Proper functioning of central nervous system (iii)DNA synthesis
Vit. C (ascorbic acid)	Fresh fruits; fresh vegetables of green variety, fresh milk, fresh meat (richest source **amla** fruit).	(i) Collagen synthesis (ii) Bone and teeth calcification (iii)Reducing agent in many chemical reactions
Vit. D	Exposure to sunlight	(i) Bone growth (ii) Calcium metabolism (iii)Acts like a hormone
Vit. E	Green leafy vegetables, vegetable oils, cereals	(i) Anti-oxidant (ii) Integrity of all membranes
Vit. K	—	—

Minerals and trace metals: A large number of minerals and trace metals are present in the body. Some of these form a part of body structural component and some others act as catalytic agents in many body reactions. Bones and skeleton are made up mainly of calcium, magnesium and phosphorus, and iron is a component of blood. Minerals like zinc, copper, manganese and magnesium are either structural part or activate a large number of enzyme systems. Iodine is a part of hormone thyroxin and triiodothyroxine. Sodium and potassium are important elements present in fluids within and outside the cells, and along with ions like chloride, bicarbonate and carbonate keep water and acid-base balance. On an average, man excretes daily 20-30 g of mineral salts consisting of Na, K, Mg, Ca, chloride, sulphate and phosphates, and this must be made good by an adequate intake of these mineral salts through our food.

Calcium : It is an essential element required for the formation and maintenance of skeleton and teeth, normal contraction of skeletal muscles, contraction of heart, nervous conduction and blood clotting. The richest source of calcium are milk (butter milk, skim milk and cheese) and green leafy vegetables.

Phosphorus: It is another important element next to calcium. Utilization of calcium is linked closely with that of phosphorus, since most of the calcium in the body is deposited as calcium phosphate in the bone and teeth. Phosphorus is also a component of nucleic acids. Phosphate esters play an important part in the cellular metabolism of other nutrients like carbohydrate, fat etc. The rich sources of phosphorus in our diets are cereals, pulses, nuts and oilseeds.

Iron : It is an essential element for the formation of haemoglobin of red blood corpuscles and plays an important role in the transport of oxygen. Tissues also require iron for various oxidation- reduction reactions. The major sources of iron are cereals, millets, pulses and green leafy vegetables. In addition to dietary iron, medicinal supplementation of iron is essential in certain specific conditions like anaemia and pregnancy.

Apart from these elements (mentioned above), a large number of other elements like sodium (Na), potassium (K) and magnesium (Mg) are essential as electrolyte to maintain the electrolyte balance. These elements are present in adequate amount in normal diet if taken in a balanced manner.

A large number of **trace elements** are required in very small amounts for a wide range of functions in the body. They are zinc (Zn), copper (Cu), selenium, cobalt, fluoride, manganese (Mn), chromium (Cr), iodine and molybdenum. Zinc is a co-factor for a number of enzymes. Copper plays an important role in iron absorption, cross-linking of connective tissues, neurotransmission and lipid metabolism. Iodine constitutes a very important part of thyroid hormone

T_3 and T_4 and plays very vital role in general body metabolism. Its deficiency causes very widespread disease 'goitre' and mental retardation. Fluoride prevents dental caries and molybdenum is involved in uric acid metabolism.

Balanced diet: Knowledge of complex interaction of nutrients, as discussed above, helps one in choosing a balanced diet as per his/her needs and in fostering the development through better nutrition. Whatever may be the diet, it should provide adequate calories to supply the body's energy needs. Carbohydrates with some fats are thus essential. Enough protein must be provided for tissue-building and repair. Besides all the necessary vitamins and minerals, the adequate diet should also provide sufficient water and enough fibre to promote good bowel function. A variety of foods, as described earlier, helps ensure that all the dietary needs of the body are met. Each of the major food groups should be represented adequately by one or more members:

(1) Cereal and grain products

(2) Milk and milk products

(3) Fruits and vegetables

(4) Legumes (beans, peas)

Yogic Diet Concept

To get success in search of health and well-being, one has to establish a dietary pattern that will sustain and promote the endeavour. Such a dietary pattern may be termed as *yogic diet*, which may be an effective tool to move ahead in that direction. It is indeed an established fact that diet has a profound effect on both body and mind, and one cannot attain complete physical and mental well-being without adequate diet.

In the concept of **'yogic diet'** all food items are classified into three categories:

1. Sattvic food
2. Rajasic food
3. Tamasic food

Sattvic food: It is the purest diet and is most suitable for yoga practitioner. It nourishes the body and maintains it in a peaceful state. It also keeps calm and purifies the mind, enabling it to function at its maximum potential. The sattvic food consists of fresh, fragrant and tasty items. It includes cereals, fresh fruits and vegetables, milk and milk products, nuts, seeds and honey.

Rajasic food: It is very hot nature, spicy, bitter, sour, pungent, dry and excessively salty. Such food items are real enemy of mind-body equilibrium. They function as body stimulant and excite the passions, making the mind restless and uncontrollable. They include fish, egg, coffee, tea, meat etc.

Tamasic food: It is stale, tasteless more or less spoiled food, and containing foul odour, artificial additives, which is at all not useful to nourish either body or mind. They make the body dull, lazy, drowsy and reduce our immune power, filling the mind with dark emotions such as anger and greed. Tamasic food items include alcohol, tobacco, onions, garlic and fermented foods such as vinegar.

Thus, while practising yoga, and to maintain the state of clarity of thought, decision making, and intellectual and contemplative thinking, and to increase the body-mind vitality, one should adopt and eat sattvic food. One should 'eat to live, not live to eat'.

SECTION II

METHODOLOGIES OF YOGA AND PREKSHA MEDITATION

- Yogic exercises 66
- Shat kriyas 81
- Asanas 95
- Mudra and bandh 125
- Kayotsarga (relaxation) 135
- Pranayama 143
- Preksha meditation 155

YOGIC EXERCISES

- For head 67
- For eyes 67
- For ears 70
- For mouth cavity 71
- For neck 72
- For shoulders 73
- For arms 74
- For chest 75
- For waist 75
- For ankle and toes 77
- For knees 78
- For spinal cord 79

Yogic Exercises

Exercise 1: *For Head*

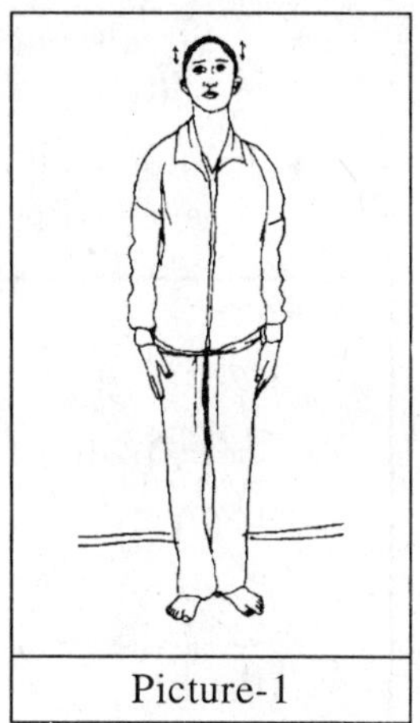
Picture-1

- Stand in erect and straight posture.
- Keep both the feet together.
- Keep both the arms hanging down and touching the thighs.
- Concentrate on forehead with eyeballs upwards.
- Contract and relax the muscles of forehead alternately.
- Repeat this times.

Exercise 2: *For Eyes*

Exercise for eyes can be performed both in erect or sitting postures, and in different stages as mentioned below. After each exercise the eyes should be closed and rested for at least 30 seconds.

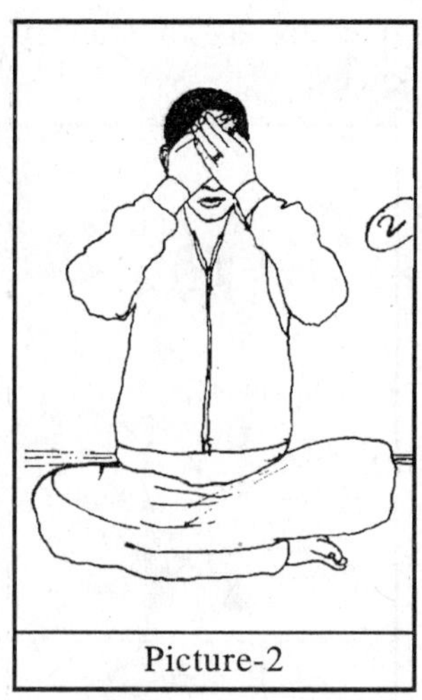
Picture-2

Stage-I

- Sit in **Sukhasana** or **Padm-asana**.
- Close the eyes and face the sun.
- Rub the palms of the hands together until they become hot.
- Place the palms over the eyes very softly.
- Remove the hands after 2 minutes.
- Keep the eyes closed throughout.
- Repeat the exercise 5 times.

Stage-II

- Assume a sitting posture.
- Strech out both the legs straight in front of the body.
- Strech out both the arms straight at the shoulder level with the thumbs pointing upwards.

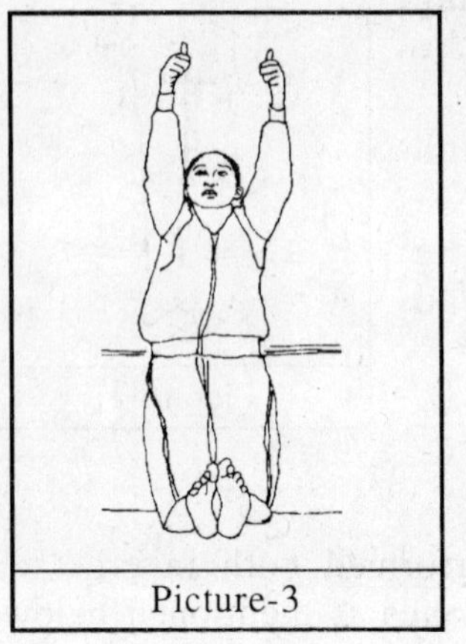

Picture-3

- Focus the eyes, without moving the head, on the following, alternately:
  - (i) left thumb while inhaling;
  - (ii) space between eyebrows while exhaling;
  - (iii) right thumb while inhaling;
  - (iv) space between eyebrows while exhaling;
- Repeat this exercise 10 times.

Stage-III

- Maintain the same sitting posture as in stage-II, with the hands resting on knees.
- Move the eyeballs upwards towards the forehead, while inhaling, looking at sky.
- Then look straight while exhaling.
- Bring down the eyeballs, while inhaling, looking at the feet.
- Repeat the process 10 times.

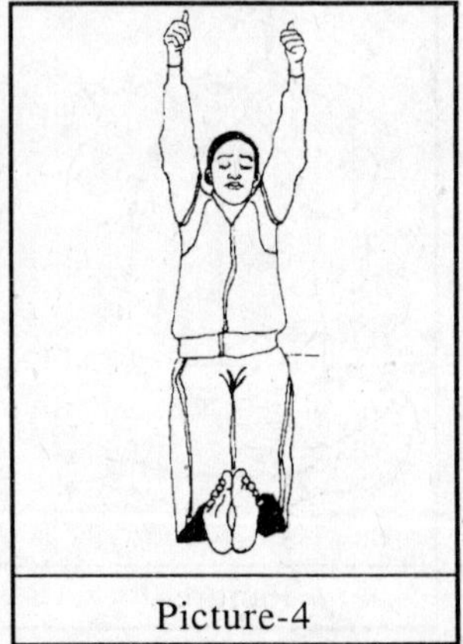

Picture-4

Stage-IV

- Maintain the same sitting posture as in stage-III.
- Inhale and hold the breath.
- Rotate the eyeballs in a circle from left to right, with the help of right thumb (make a circular movement with the right thumb while keeping the eyes focused on the thumb).
- Exhale.
- Inhale and hold the breath.
- Then rotate the eyeballs in a circle from right to left similarly.
- Exhale.
- Then keep the eyes closed and rest for 30 seconds.

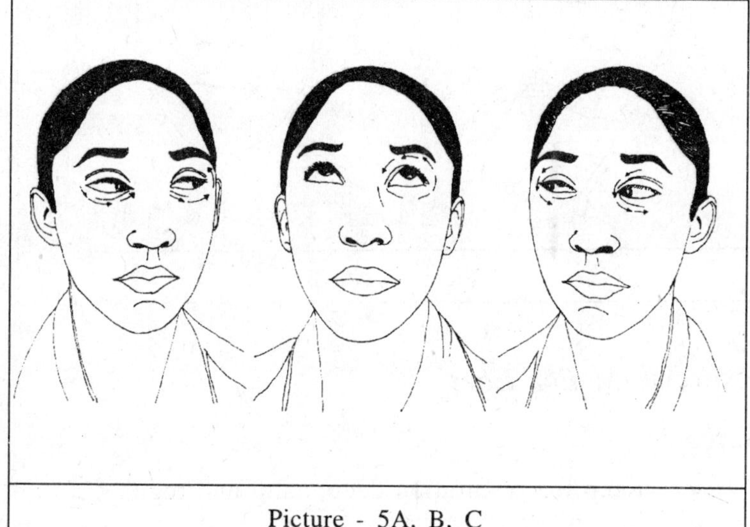

Picture - 5A, B, C

Stage-V

- Maintain the same posture as in stage-IV.
- Inhale and hold the breath.
- Focus the eyes on a distant object without blinking the eyelids.
- Exhale.
- Inhale and hold the breath.
- Focus the eyes on the nose, while sinking the eyelids.
- Exhale.
- Repeat it 5 times.

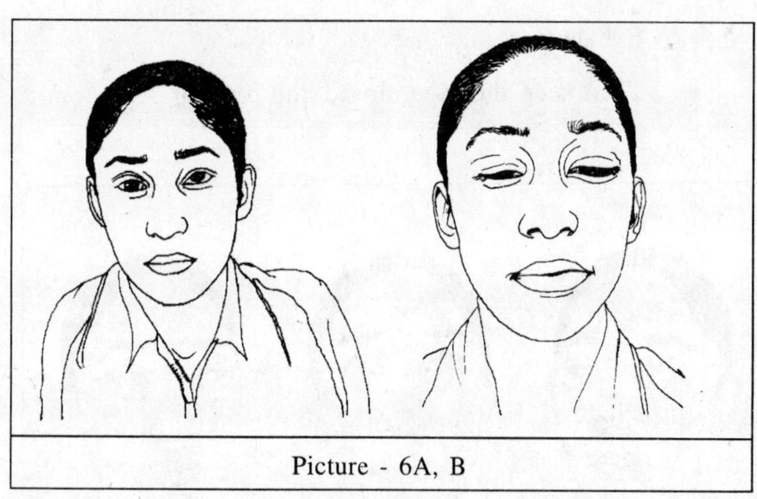

Picture - 6A, B

Exercise 3: *For Ears*

Stage-I

- Keep the respiration deep, calm and regular.
- Rub the palms together until they become hot.

- Place them over the ears of their respective side.
- Press them to listen very peculiar inner sound.

Stage-II

- Insert the respective index finger in the ears and rotate them with gentle pressure.

Stage-III

- Massage the pinna of external ear by pulling it gently upward and downward.

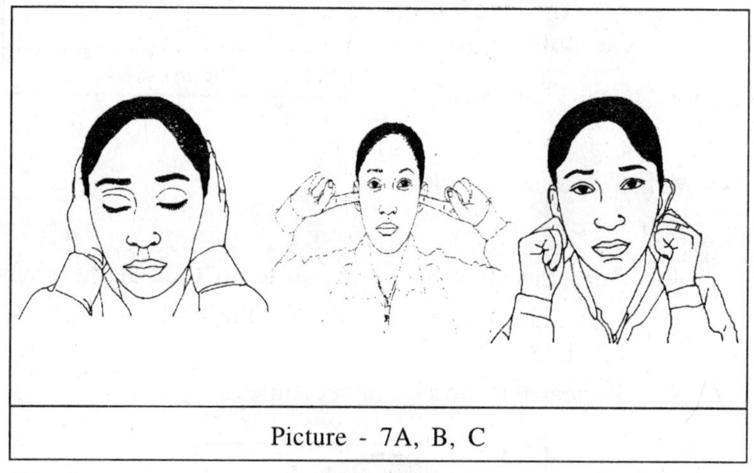

Picture - 7A, B, C

Exercise 4: *For Mouth Cavity*

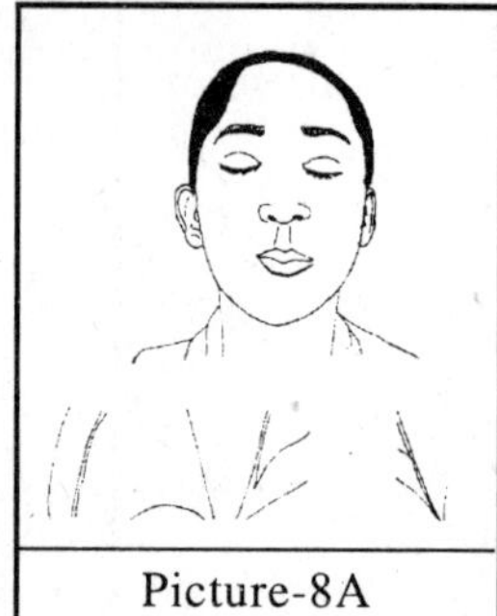

Picture-8A

Stage-I

- Open the mouth and fill the mouth cavity with air, keeping the cheeks inflated.
- Repeat it three times.

Stage-II

- First bring the teeth and jaws together with full pressure.
- Then open fingers of either of the hands inside the mouth cavity and produce any typical but rhythmic sound like A.A.A.A....., for the maximum possible duration.
- Repeat it thrice.

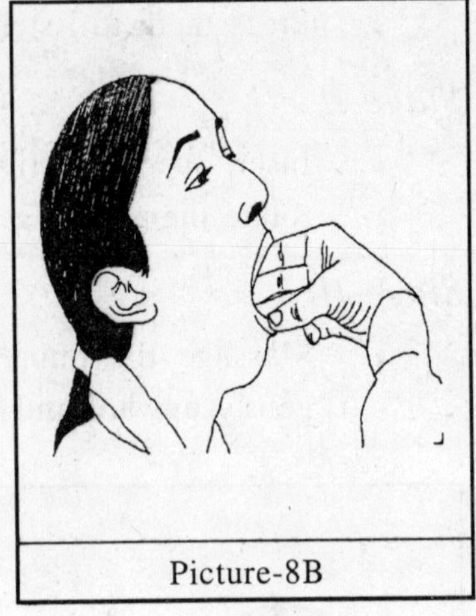

Picture-8B

Exercise 5: *For Neck*

Stage-I

- Turn the neck backward so as to look at the sky.
- Bring down the neck so that the chin touches the clavicle.
- Repeat this process three times.

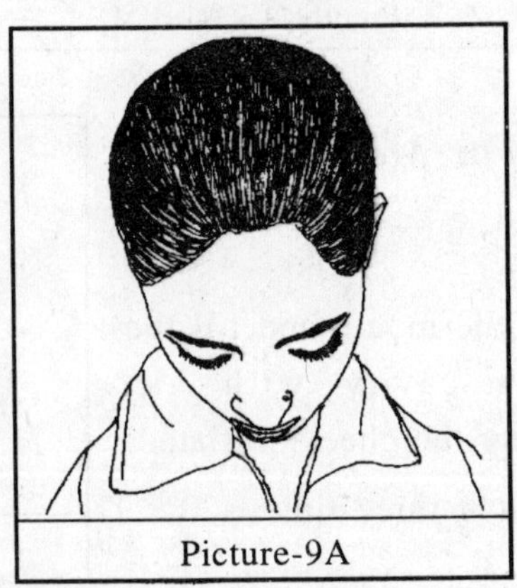

Picture-9A

Stage-II

- Turn the neck towards the right and left shoulder, touching it alternately.
- Repeat it five times.

Stage-III

- Rotate the neck clockwise and anticlockwise alternately, very slowly and gently.
- Repeat it three times.

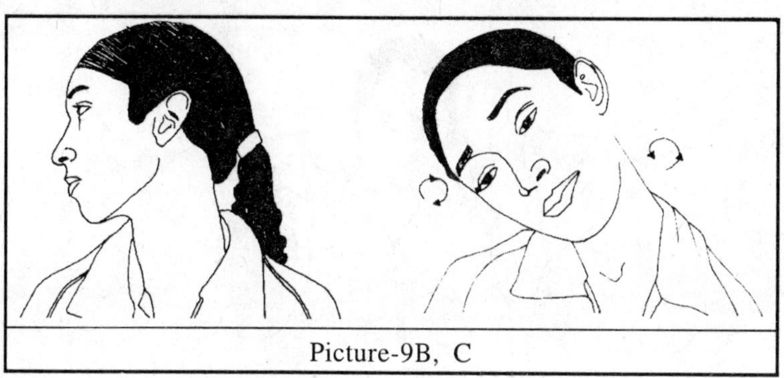

Picture-9B, C

Exercise 6: *For Shoulders*

Stage-I

- Stand erect and straight.
- Keep the arms hanging straight with fists closed.
- Raise both the shoulders up while inhaling.
- Bring them down while exhaling.
- Repeat it five times.

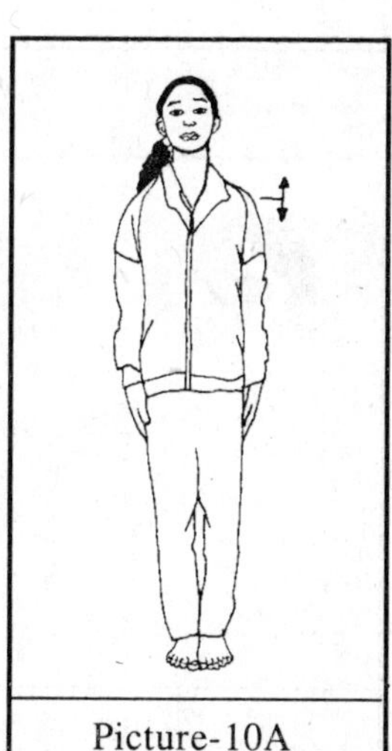

Picture-10A

Stage-II

- Maintain the same posture.
- Bend both the arms towards shoulders with the fingers touching them.
- Rotate the folded arms from their shoulder joints, tilting forward and backward, in clockwise and anticlockwise direction.
- Repeat the exercise five times.

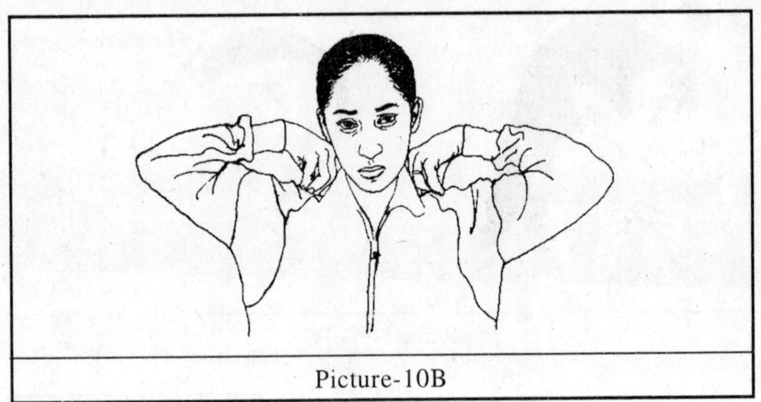

Picture-10B

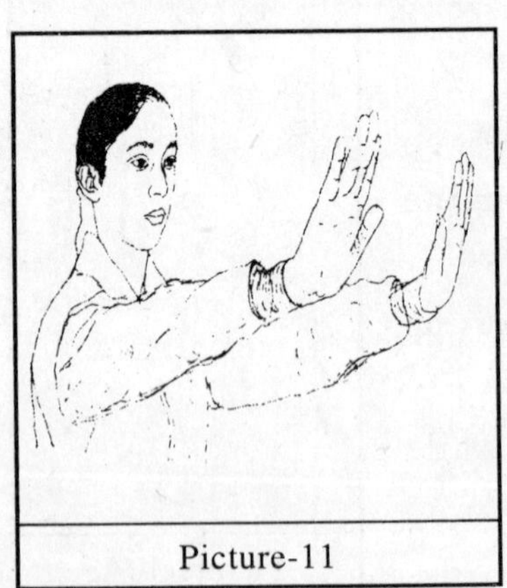

Picture-11

Exercise 7: *For Arms*

- Stand in erect posture.
- Stretch the arms forward.
- Move the fingers up and down — 10 times.
- Now move the palm along with fingers up and down from wrist joints — 10 times.

- Now fold the arms inside from elbow joint — 5 times.
- Then strech the arms straight and rotate them from shoulder joint gently in clockwise and anticlockwise direction — 5 times.

Exercise 8: *For Chest*

- Inhale for full chest expansion.
- Strech the arms forward and fold the fingers like lion's paw, and exhale.
- Bring the arms back towards chest with next breath (inhale) and with full force like pulling a rope in a tug of war.
- Now spread the arms from chest to shoulder.
- Repeat this three times.

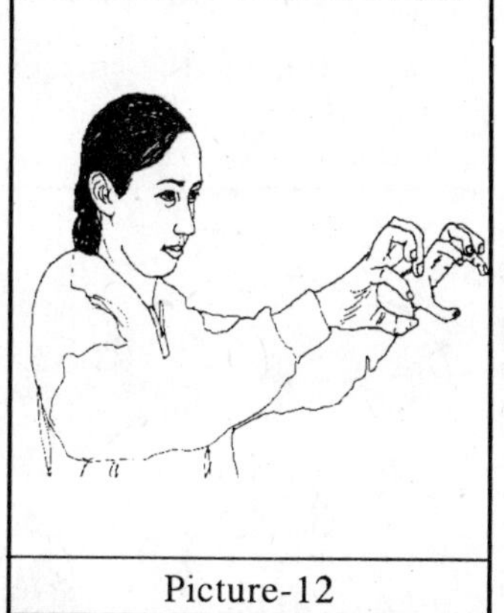

Picture-12

Exercise 9: *For Waist*

Stage-I

- Maintain the erect posture.
- Raise both hands upwards with forceful streching while inhaling.
- Now bend forward and try to touch the knees by forehead; the fingers of hands should touch the toes of the feet, while exhaling.

- Now return to the erect position with hand raised upward, while inhaling, and then bend backward.
- Do it thrice gently, slowly and carefully.

Stage-II

- Maintain the erect posture.
- Raise the right hand up and keep the left hand with left knee.
- Stretch the right hand towards left over the head and bend towards left from waist position.
- Repeat the process from the other side also.

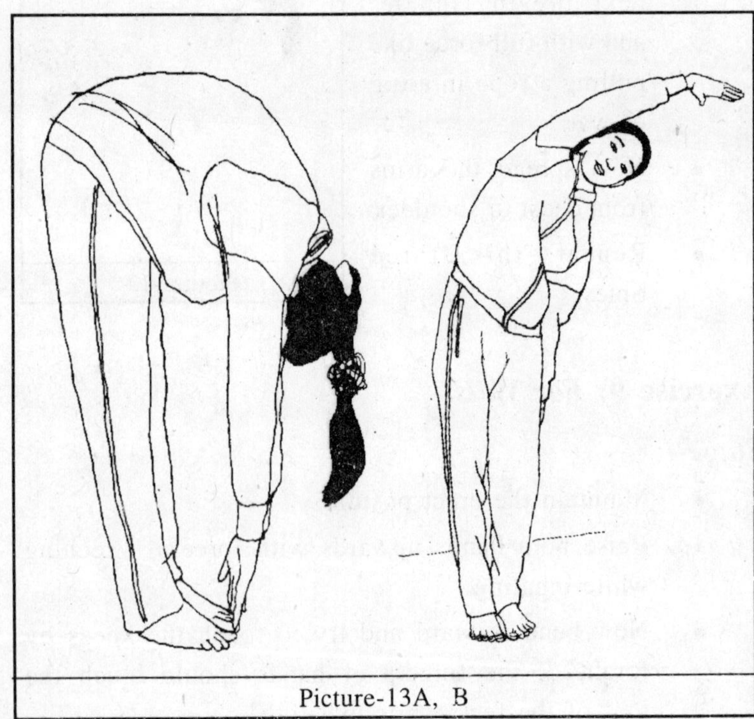

Picture-13A, B

Exercise 10: *For Ankle and Toes*

- Assume the sitting posture with legs stretched in front of the body.
- Draw the hands in the back of body by the side of the trunk.
- Lean a little towards backside with the support of straight arms.
- Move the toes of both feet slowly backward and forward, keeping the feet stationary — 10 times.
- Now move both feet forward and backward, bending them from ankle joint — 10 times.
- Now rotate the right and left feet simultaneously about the ankle, both in clockwise and anticlockwise direction — 10 times each.

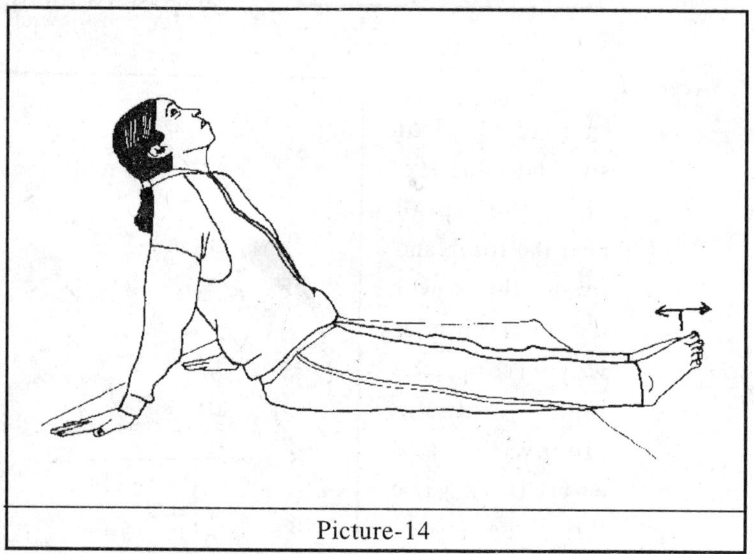

Picture-14

Exercise 11: *For Knees*

Stage-I

- Assume a sitting posture.
- Bend the right leg from the knee joint and put the hands under right thigh.

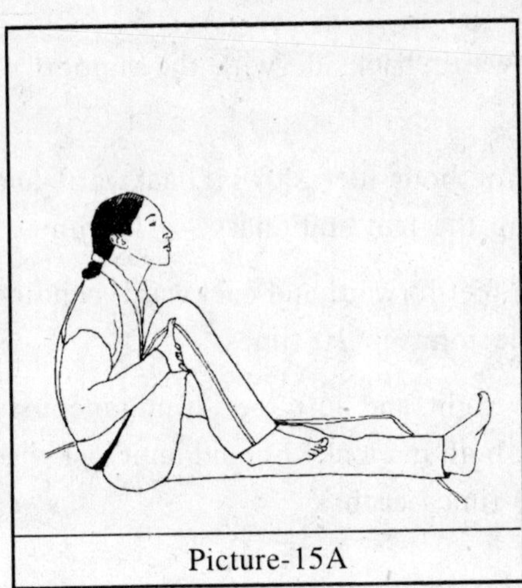
Picture-15A

- Stretch the right leg forward without allowing the heel or toe to touch the ground.
- Then fold the right leg maximum possible from the knee joint, bringing the heel near the right buttock.
- Repeat the process at least 10 times.

Stage-II

- Instead of stretching the leg, hold the thigh near the trunk and rotate the lower leg in a circular way from the knee joint, in clockwise and anticlockwise directions.

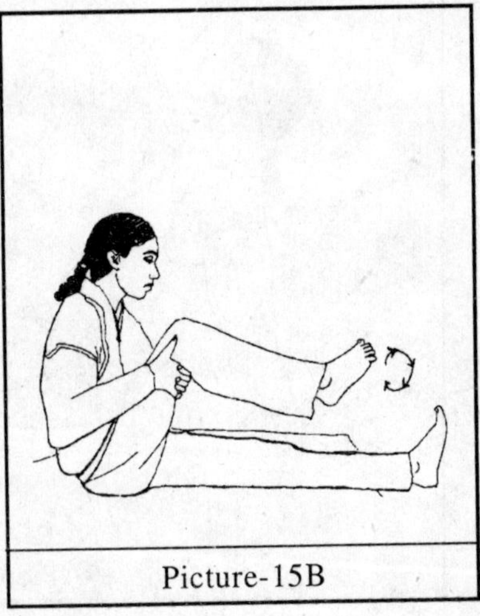
Picture-15B

- Remain in the same posture.
- Repeat the same process with both the legs 10 times each.

Stage-III

- Remain in the same sitting posture.
- Fold the right leg and place the right foot on the left thigh.
- Hold the right foot with left hand and place the right hand over the knee.
- Rotate the right knee in a circle 10 times.
- Repeat the process with left knee also.

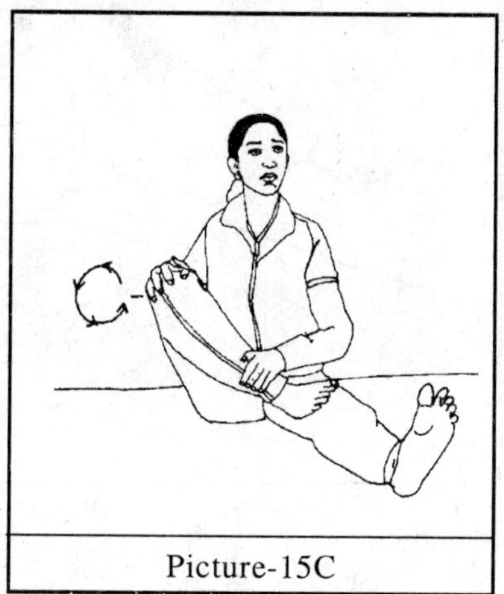

Picture-15C

Exercise 12: *For Spinal Cord*

- Adopt the sitting posture.
- Keep both the legs streched in front and keeping the maximum possible distance between them.
- Stretch the right hand to touch the left toe and left hand fully stretched in the back side.
- Try to keep both the hands in a straight line.

- Now turn the head looking backward at the thumb of left hand.
- Repeat the same process by other direction.
- Do it slowly and gently five times each.

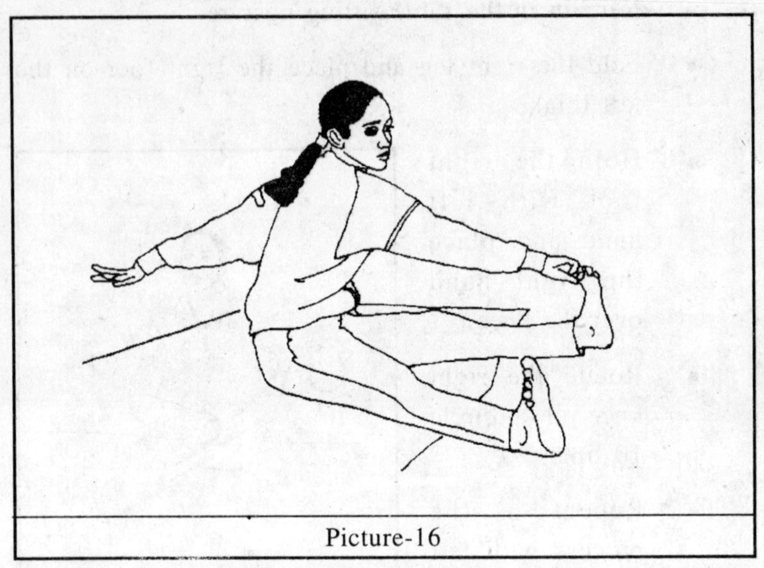

Picture-16

:::::::::

SHAT KRIYAS

- Neti 82
- Dhauti 84
- Kunjal 86
- Nauli 88
- Basti 89
- Kapal Bhati 90
- Trataka 92

Shat Kriyas

Yoga science gives equal emphasis to a few cleansing processes, as it does to asanas and pranayama. To gain maximum benefit from yoga exercises, cleansing of the body systems is essential. Without eliminating toxins and impurities from within the body, the effects of appropriate yoga exercises are not ensured. Ancient yoga masters have described six scientific yoga techniques known as **'Shat karmas'** or **'Shat kriyas'** to get body cleansing. These techniques are not only important from normal physical and mental health point of view, but also they are much valuable in healing several psychosomatic disorders. The following six purificatory exercises (kriyas) constitute the Shat kriyas.

1. Neti
2. Dhauti
3. Nauli
4. Basti
5. Kapal bhati
6. Tratak

Neti

Neti is a process that clears and cleans the nasal passage. This includes Jal Neti and Sutra Neti.

Procedure of Jal neti: It is a process of cleaning the nasal passage with the help of saline water.

- Fill the Jal Neti pot with lukewarm saline water.

- Insert the spout of Jal neti pot into left nostril after tilting the head towards right.
- Keep the mouth open, and breathe through mouth.
- Pour gently the water from Jal neti pot and let it flow in through the left nostril and out through right one.
- Allow the water to flow through the nostrils for about 30 seconds.
- Remove the spout of neti pot from the nose.
- Repeat the same process from right nostril but keeping the head tilted towards left.
- After completing the process, fully clean and dry the nostrils.

Procedure of Sutra neti:

- Take a catheter or 12 inches (30 cm) piece of cotton string stiffened with wax.
- Pass the catheter into one nostril and pull it through the mouth to and fro very gently.
- Do it 20-40 times.
- Now remove the catheter from nostril and repeat the process with other nostril.

Caution: Do it under strict guidance.

Dhauti

It is a general body cleansing technique. There are four kinds of Dhautis, which clear away the impurities of body. These are :

- Antar dhauti: internal cleansing
- Danta dhauti: cleaning the teeth
- Hrid dhauti: cleaning the rectum
- Mool shodhana: cleaning the rectum.

However, the following dhauti kriyas are in common practice.

Vastra dhauti:

- Take a fine and specially prepared cotton cloth, 2 inches (5 cm) broad and more than 14 ft (5 m) long.
- Insert one end of the cloth in the mouth.
- start swallowing it slowly and carefully, while sipping a little amount of warm water.
- The cloth is drawn down bit by bit.
- Try to swallow maximum length of cloth.
- Then, after a few minutes (4-5 minutes), pull it out gently to remove accumulated mucous and water from the stomach and oesophagus.
- At first one may feel nauseous and may succeed in swallowing only an inch (2.5 cm) or two, but after some practice one may swallow the full length of cloth.

Caution: This exercise should be done in strict supervision of a qualified yoga teacher.

Varisara dhauti or Shankha prakshalan: This technique is termed shankha prakshalan because it washes the Conch-shaped intestine.

- Take sufficient amount of lukewarm saline water.
- Drink 2-3 glasses of that water.
- Then practice Tadasana, Tiryak tadasana, Kati-chakrasana, Tiryak bhujangasana and Udar akarshan asana. (each asana — 5 times)
- Drink another 2 glasses of saline (salty) water and again practice those asanas.
- Again drink 2 glasses of water followed by those asanas.
- Go to the toilet to clear the bowel without any strain.
- Come out of the toilet, again drink 2 glasses of salty water, practice the five same asanas and go to the toilet.
- Continue this process till you get your alimentary canal completely cleaned.
- Total consumption of water to clear the bowel varies from person to person. It may require drinking of 20-25 glasses of water.

Caution: No solid or liquid food material should be taken prior to the process.

- It is a long process and should not be done without proper guidance of a trained yoga teacher.

Agnisar kriya or Vahnisar dhauti:

- Assume the posture of Vajrasana, keeping distance between knees but both toes together.
- Keep the hands on knees, arms straight.
- Open the mouth and take out the tongue.
- Start breathing rapidly and pressing in the navel knot towards spine at least 100 times, by contracting and expanding the abdomen. This process of abdomen movement and respiration resembles the panting of a dog.
- In the advanced form of Agnisar kriya, maintaining the same Vajrasana posture, exhale fully, retain the breath and perform Jalandhara bandh. Then contract and expand abdominal muscles rapidly so long you are able to retain the breath.

Vaman dhauti: In this process vomiting is induced by tickling the back of throat. It is also known as **Kunjal kriya**.

- Prepare some salty water.
- Drink maximum quantity of this water, as much as you can, in standing posture.
- Then lean forward and place the middle and index fingers of the right hand in mouth,

extending them up to throat as deep as possible. Press the back portion of tongue.

- This will initiate the strong urge of vomiting and water will come out of mouth.
- Continue pressing the tongue till the stomach is empty.

Dand dhauti: In this process the food pipe, oesophagus, is cleaned, from throat to stomach, by inserting a specially prepared stick, may be made up of banana-tree stem, in the size of half an inch (1.25 cm) in diameter and two and half inches (6.5 cm) long.

- Carefully insert the stick into oesophagus till its lower portion reaches the stomach. Then take it out very slowly.

Caution: It is a delicate exercise and involves severe risk; and hence it should not be done without an expert's direction and supervision.

Danta-moola dhauti: Rub the teeth (gums) with catechu powder or with pure earth or with the help of adequate toothpaste and brush, until all dental impurities are removed.

The really important thing is the intelligent and persistent massaging of the gums and not so much the brushing of the teeth, which in fact produces the opposite effect.

Jivha-shodhan dhauti :

- Join the index, middle and ring fingers together, place them into the throat, and slowly rub well the root of the tongue, and wash out. Expel the phlegm.
- Rub the tongue with butter and milk, repeatedly. Then by carefully holding the tip of the tongue, pull it out gradually and slowly.

The rubbing of the root of the tongue prevents the accumulation of phlegm which occurs throughout the years, and which is responsible for stale breath and general lack of freshness in one's mouth; it keeps at bay throat infections, even tooth decay. The manipulation (milking) of the tongue stimulates the inner recesses of the oral cavity and greatly adds to the perfect functioning of various glands in the deep of neck, i.e. thyroid and parathyroids.

Nauli

It is a yogic technique of massaging the whole abdomen and stomach by contracting and rolling the abdominal muscles, specially the rectus abdominis muscle.

- Stand erect with the feet separate by metre.
- Lean forward and place the hand on both thighs just above the knees.
- Perform Uddiyan bandh.
- Now contract the muscles rectus abdominis and isolate them at the centre of the abdomen (Stage-I: Madhyama nauli).

- Now bring the rectus abdominis muscles at the left side of the abdomen (Stage-II: Vama nauli).
- Now bring the rectus abdominis muscles at the right side of abdomen (Stage-III: Dakshina nauli).
- Now try to roll the rectus abdominis muscles so that they move from left of centre and then to right, while holding the breath outside (Stage-IV).
- Then inhale, relax and after normal respiration again repeat the process of rolling the muscles in opposite direction, i.e. right to left.

Basti

It is a hath yoga process of yogic enema to clean the colon by sucking in air or water through anus. There are two types of basti:

- Jal basti
- Sthal basti

Jal basti:

- Stand erect in water up to navel, preferably in free flowing river water.
- Lean forward and place the hands on the knees.
- Perform Uddiyan bandh, and expand the anal sphincter.
- Draw the water into the bowel for some time and then expel it forcefully through anus.
- Jal basti can also be performed by sitting in cool, fresh water up to navel and by adopting Ashwini mudra.

Sthal basti :

- Assume the sitting pose of Paschimottanasana.
- Adopt ashwini mudra for at least 25-30 times, sucking air into bowel through anus.
- Retain it for some time and then expel it through anus.

Kapal Bhati

Kapal bhati is basically a technique of pranayama. Some ancient yogic scriptures have also classified it as a part of Shat karmas. It has great resemblance with Bhastrika pranayama. The practice of Kapal bhati not only purifies the frontal area of brain, but also gives adequate massage to the abdominal organs and improves respiration. It is of three types:

(a) Vatkrama

(b) Vyutkrama

(c) Sheetkrama

Vatkrama:

- Sit in an easy posture, say Sukhasana.
- Hold the back straight upright.
- Close the eyes.
- Relax the body.
- Breathe in through the left nostril.
- Breathe out through the right nostril.
- Then breathe in through right nostril.
- Breathe out through left nostril.

This inspiration and expiration should be effortless. All disorders of the phlegm are destroyed by this practice.

Vyutkrama :

- Maintain the same sitting posture.
- Draw water through both nostrils.
- Expel the water through mouth very slowly.

It cleans and clears the nasal cavity by removing mucus from the passage and cavity.

Sheetkrama:

- Maintain the sitting posture.
- Suck water noisily through the mouth.
- Expel the water through the nostrils with a sneezing sound.

This practice enhances the immune capacity of the body and destroy all types of phyelgm disorders.

Note: The cleansing of the frontal sinus is done through Kapalbhati by both 'dry' or 'wet' method. Proper care should be taken while performing the wet practice. One has to make sure that there is sufficient air in the lungs to cope with any unexpected emergency, i.e. in case some of the water finds its way into the air passages, so that it may be easily expelled. The water should be warm with a little lemon juice in it, to improve the prophylactic aspect of such practices. The 'dry' practice serves as preparation for the exercises of pranayama, apart from inherent therapeutic virtues. It purifies the Nadis (subtle channels of cosmic energy — Prana) and establishes a gentle rhythm throughout the whole organism.

Trataka

The practice of trataka involves gazing at a point or at a particular object without blinking the eyes at all. In other words it is a process of focusing the eyes at a point and in turn to concentrate the mind also at that particular point. The point of gazing and concentration may be external (outside the body) or internal, while maintaining self awareness. Gazing outside the body is called **bahir tratak** and internal gazing is known as **anter tratak**. Practice of this technique yields the enhanced attention capacity, concentration power and latent potential of mind. In ancient yoga text, *Gherand Samhita* it is classified as one of the Shat karmas. While the other five components of Shat karmas are related with cleansing of the body, the trataka acts as a bridge between physical exercises and mental practices, leading to internal awareness.

Procedure :

- Assume a meditative asana posture in cool, least lighted room.
- Light a candle and place it on a small bench at the level of eyes at a distance of 2 feet (60 cm) from the eyes.
- Relax the body, close the eyes and keep the body like a statue with straight spine.
- Allow no movement at all throughout the practice.
- Now open the eyes and gaze at the brightest top of the flame without movement of eyeballs or blinking.
- Continue to gaze at the flame with full concentration and consciousness, and without any awareness of the rest of the body.
- Initially gaze for 2-3 minutes.
- Then close your eyes.
- Try to visualize the after-image of the candle flame in front of closed eyes.
- When this after-image disappears, open the eyes and again start gazing the flame tip.
- Increase the duration of gazing each time and do it for maximum possible duration.

Tratak can also be practised on a small point, finger tip, nosetip, a shadow, the full moon or any shining object. Duration of the practice may be increased up to 20 minutes, but in the beginning undue strain should not be taken.

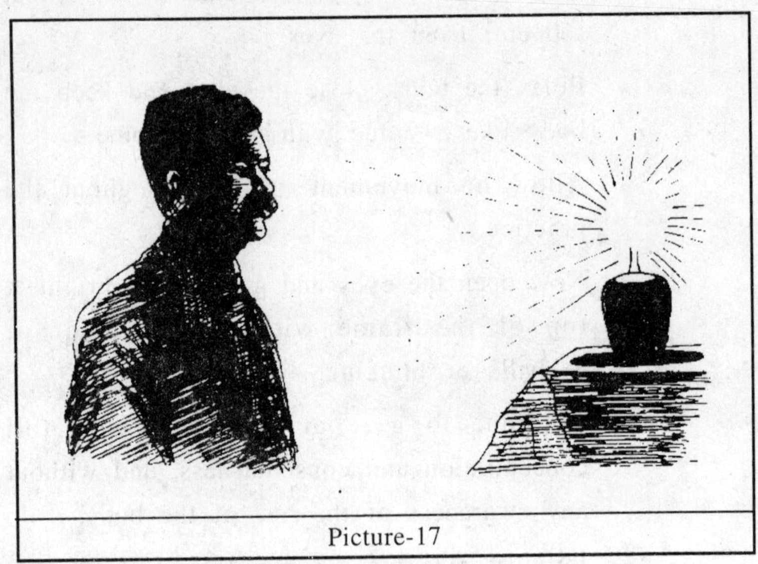

Picture-17

———:::::::::———

ASANAS

- Surya Namaskar 96
- Tadasana 103
- Vrikshasana 103
- Trikonasana 104
- Kati Chakrasana 105
- Padmasana 106
- Sukhasana 106
- Simhasana 107
- Vajrasana 108
- Supta Vajrasana 108
- Ushtrasana 109
- Bhujangasana 110
- Shalabhasana 111
- Dhanurasana 111
- Makarasana 112
- Uttan padasana 113
- Pawan muktasana 114
- Halasana 115
- Matsyasana 116
- Paschimottanasana 116
- Ardha Matsyendrasana 117
- Naukasana 119
- Siddhasana 120
- Sarvangasana 121
- Vipareet karni 122
- Shirshasana 122
- Shavagasana 124

Asanas

Surya Namaskar (Sun Salutation)

Surya Namaskar makes the whole body supple for doing yogic asanas efficiently. It comprises 12 graceful positions. Each position supplements and counteracts the one before in succession, stretching the body in a different way and alternately contracting and expanding the chest to regulate the breathing. It brings about remarkable flexibility to the muscles, joints and spine, along with massaging all the internal organs. One round of 12 positions is to be performed in two sequences. In the beginning start slowly and do it in succession.

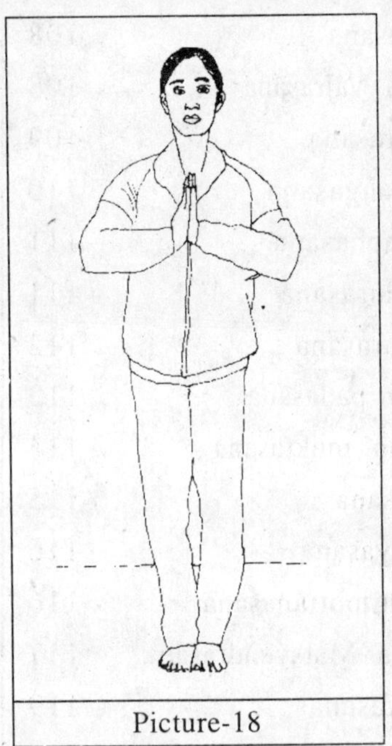

Picture-18

Position-I

- Stand erect with feet together.
- Keep the palms in prayer position in front of the chest.
- Relax the body and exhale.

Position-II

- Inhale.
- While inhaling, raise the arms over head, separated by shoulder width.

- Arch back the head and upper trunk from the waist.
- Keep legs straight.

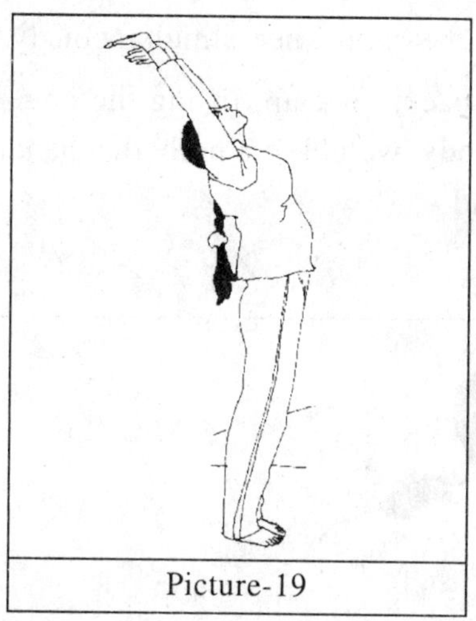

Picture-19

Position-III

- While exhaling, bend forward, bringing the palms down and touching the ground on either side of the feet.
- Keep the legs straight.
- Try to touch the knees with forehead, but do not strain unnecessarily (in the beginning slightly bend the knees if required).

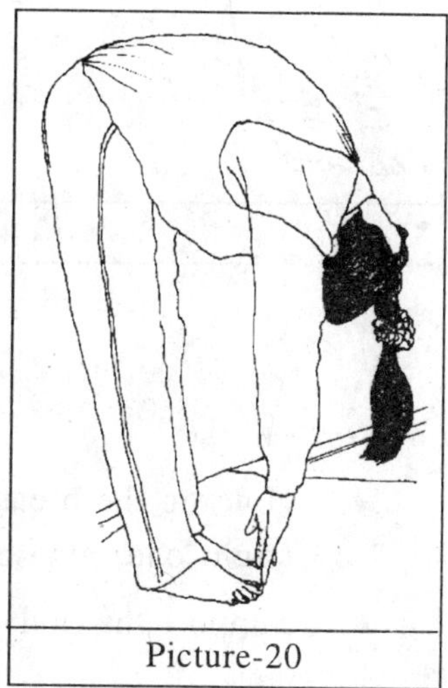

Picture-20

Position-IV

- Inhale.
- Stretch the left leg back and place the knee on the floor. Keep the arms straight.
- Bend the right knee simultaneously.
- Arch back, look up, lifting the chin and putting all the body weight on both the hands touching the ground.

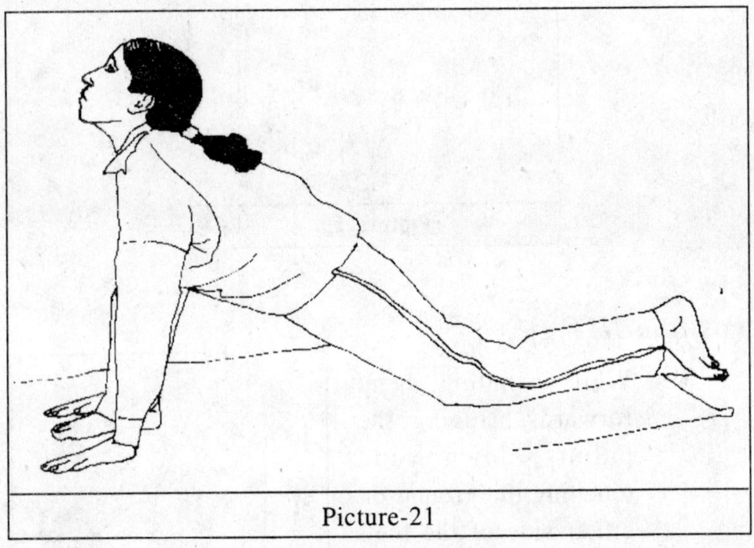

Picture-21

Position-V

- Holding the breath inside, bring back the other leg (right one) also beside the left leg.
- Support the body weight on hands and toes.

- Keep the head and body in one straight line and look at ground between the hands.
- Exhale while stretching the right leg.

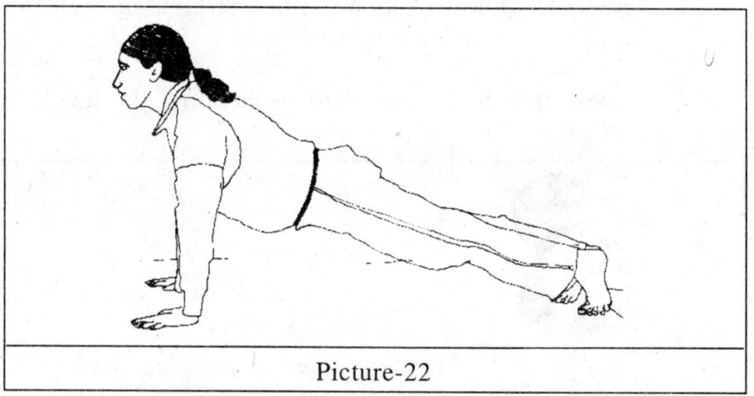

Picture-22

Position-VI

- Hold the breath outside.
- Lower the body downwards so that both feet, both knees, the chest, palm of the hands and chin touch the ground.
- The hip and abdomen should be a little up from the ground and toes should be curled inward.

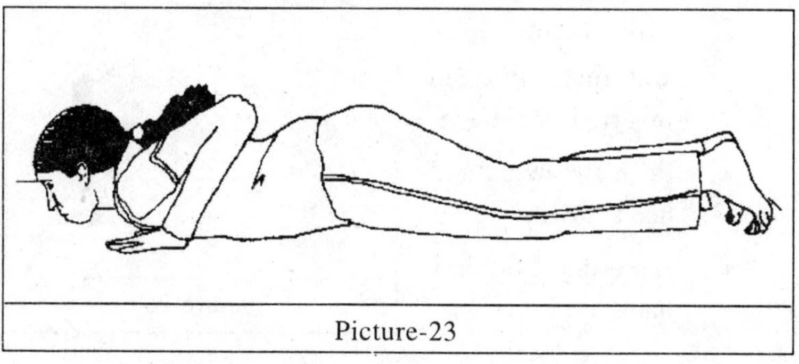

Picture-23

Position-VII

- Inhale.
- Lower the hips.
- Raise the body from waist and straighten both the arms.
- Look up a little backward by bending the head.

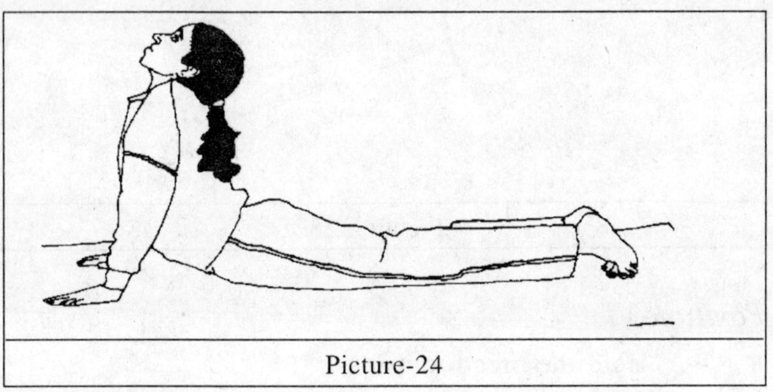

Picture-24

Position-VIII

- Exhale.
- Curl your toes under.
- Raise youp hips and pivot into an inverted 'V' shape.
- Push the heels and head down.
- Keep the shoulders back.

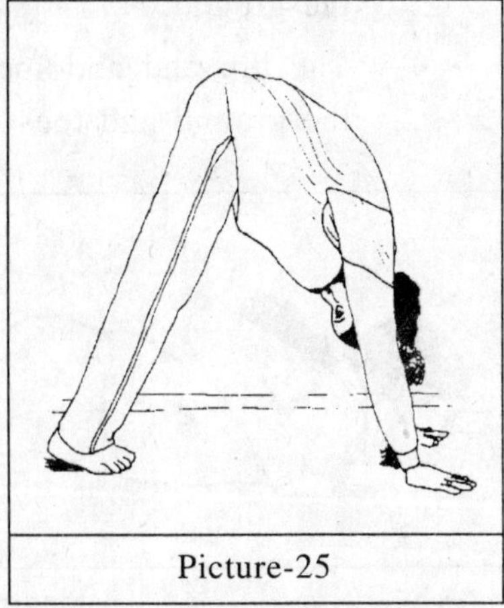

Picture-25

Position-IX

- Inhale.
- Step forward and place the left leg between the hands.
- Rest the right knee on the ground.
- Arch back and look up towards sky as in Position-IV.

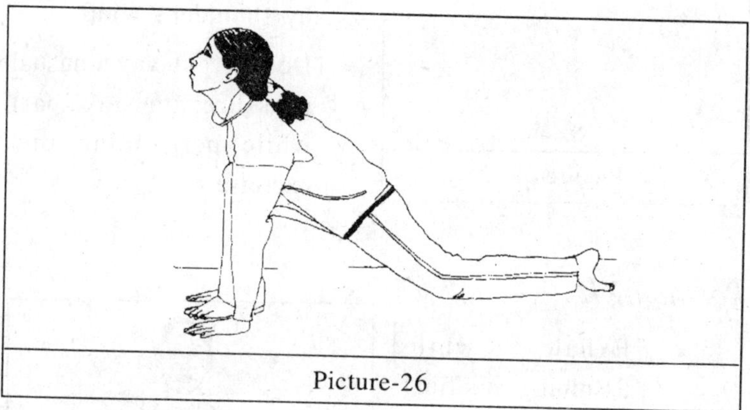

Picture-26

Position-X

- Exhale.
- Put the right and left legs, straightening both of them.
- Try to bring the forehead closer to knees without excess strain.
- Keep both the palms on ground.

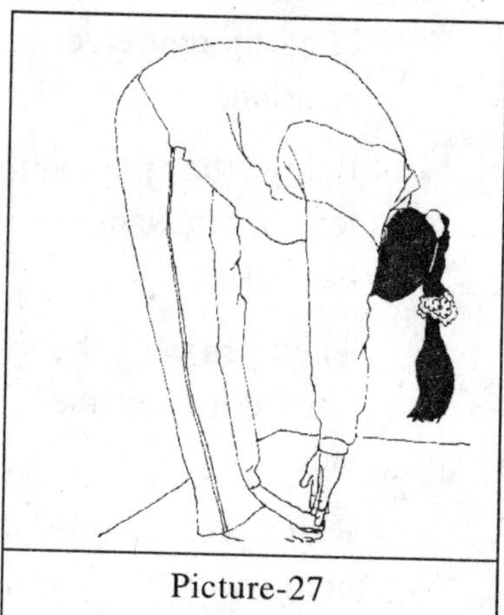

Picture-27

Position-XI

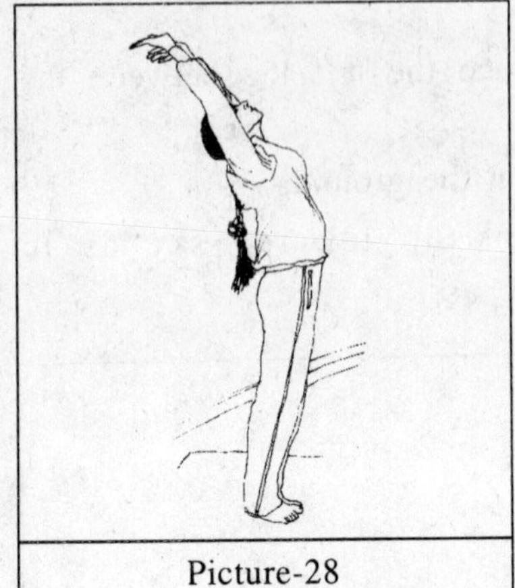
Picture-28

- Inhale.
- Stretch the arms towards back over the head and bend back from the waist very slowly and gently.
- Keep the arms separated by shoulder's width.
- Do not put any unusual pressure on any part while performing this exercise.

Position-XII

- Exhale while assuming this final position.
- Gently come back to an upright erect position.
- Bring the plams together in Namaskar pose.
- Then bring the arms down by the sides.
- Relax the whole body.

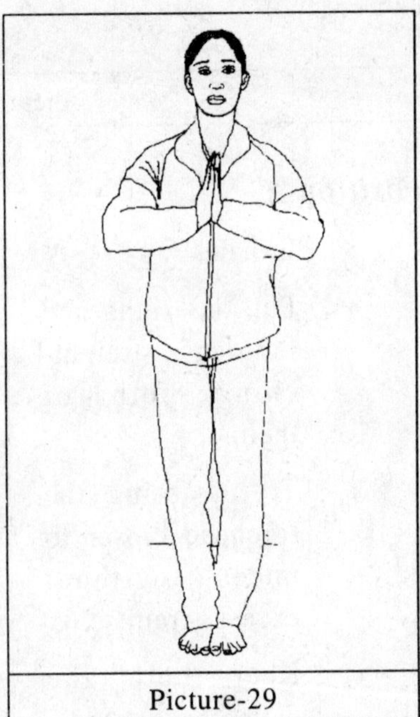
Picture-29

Tadasana

- Stand erect with the feet together, the heels and big toes touching each other.
- Raise the arms up over the head, fingers interlocked and palms facing upward.
- Keep the stomach in, chest forward.
- Now look up at the hands.
- Lift the heels and stretch the whole body upward.
- Slowly return the heels on to the ground.
- Hold the breath inside while stretching the body.
- Repeat the process five times.

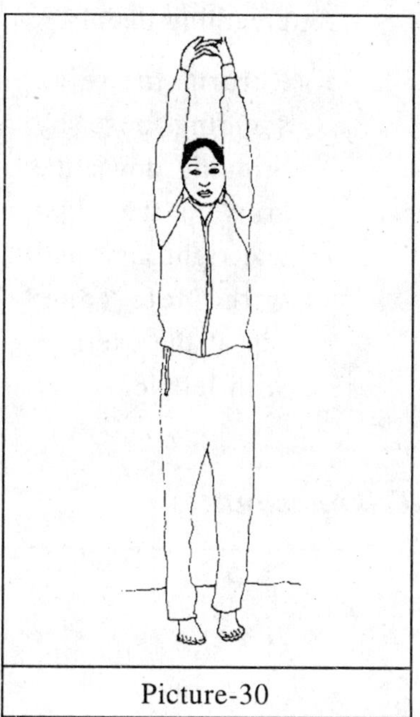

Picture-30

Vrikshasana

- Stand erect with the feet together.
- Bend the right leg from the knee and place the heel of this leg at the root of left thigh. Rest the foot on the thigh, toes pointing downward.
- Now raise the arms straight over the head, joining both the palms together in worship pose and

pointing towards sky. Balance on the left leg.

- Remain in this pose for a few seconds while breathing deeply.
- Return in relax standing pose by bringing down the arms to the sides and right leg apart with left one; repeat the exercise with left leg.

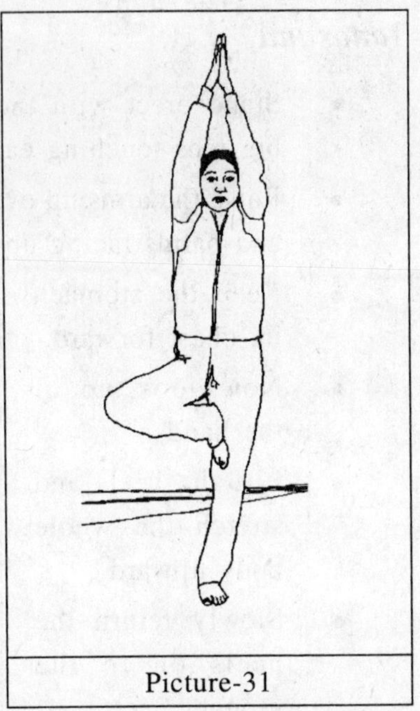

Picture-31

Trikonasana

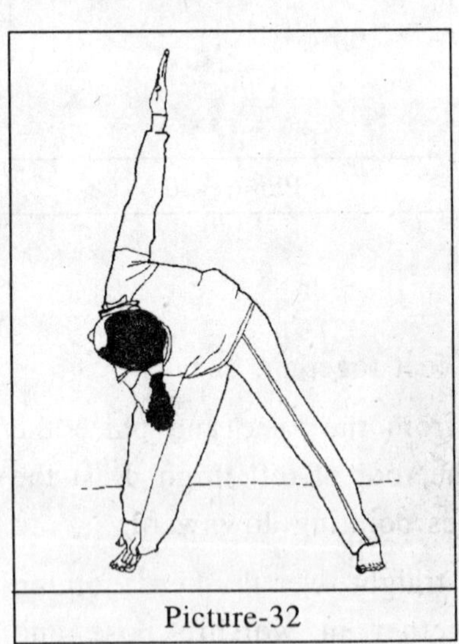

Picture-32

- Stand erect with the feet 60-90 cm apart.
- Take a deep inhalation and hold the breath inside.
- Extend both the arms sideways in line with the shoulder.
- Bend the body from the waist at 90 degrees angle.
- Look forward and touch the right toe with left hand.

- Now watch upward to the straight arm with the palm facing right.
- Remain in this posture for a few seconds, return to the easy standing posture, lowering and placing the arms in the sides, and exhale.
- Repeat the exercise with the right hand touching the left toe and left hand going up.

Kati Chakrasana

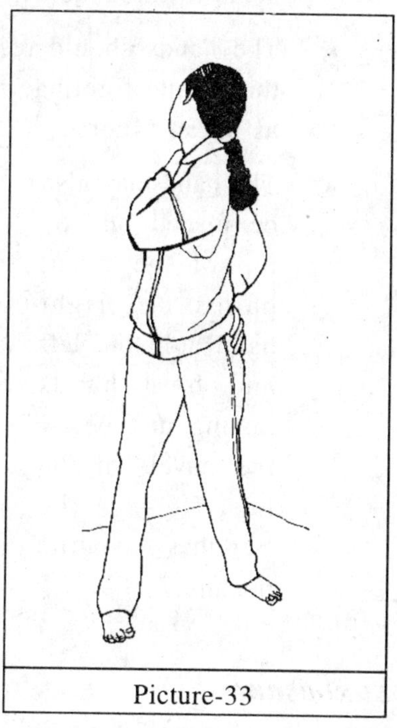
Picture-33

- Adopt a standing posture with the feet 2 feet (60 cm) apart.
- Extend both the arms straight in the line of shoulders.
- Give a twist to the upper part of the body from the waist slowly while placing the left hand on right shoulder and wrapping the right arm around the trunk, breathing normally, and rotating the head also in the same direction.
- Repeat the process by placing right hand on left shoulder and wrapping left arm around the trunk.
- Practice it at least five times.

Padmàsana

- Assume a sitting posture with legs extended forward.
- Fold the right leg and place it on left thigh.
- Then fold the left leg and place it on right thigh.
- The feet should be far enough back to touch the heels to the abdomen on either side.
- The hands should rest on the knees, palms open, thumb and forefinger jointed in the gesture known as 'Gyan Mudra'.
- The hand may also be placed one on top of the other, palms up, right hand atop the left and both hands resting just below the navel, in the lap — the Buddhas' favourite posture.

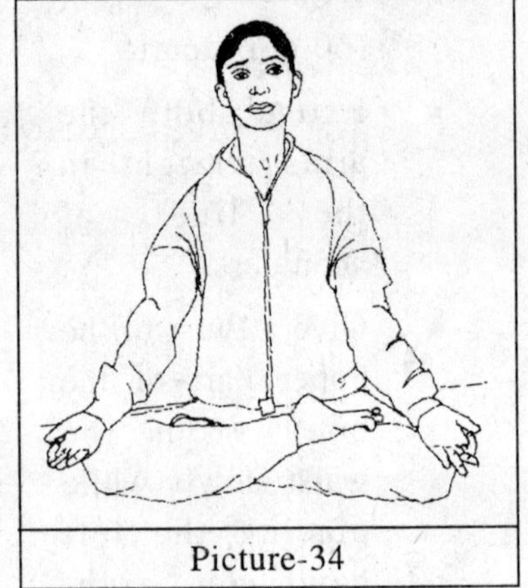

Picture-34

Sukhasana

- Assume a sitting posture with the legs extended in front of the body.
- Fold the right foot and place it under the left thigh.
- Then fold the left foot and place it under the right thigh.

- Rest the hands on the knees, palms facing downward.
- Keep the head, neck and vertebral column in a straight line.
- Eyes should remain closed.
- Maintain the posture as long as possible comfortably.

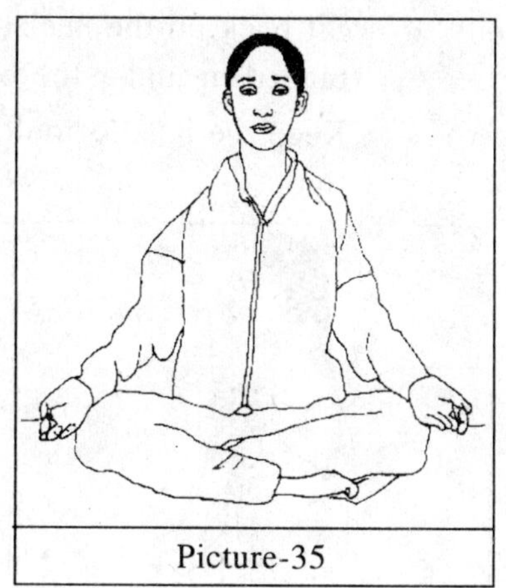
Picture-35

Simhasana

- Sit in Vajrasana posture with the knees apart, looking towards sun.
- Place the hands between the knees, palms on the floor and fingers pointing backward.
- Lean a little forward, putting the weight of the body on both the straightened hands.

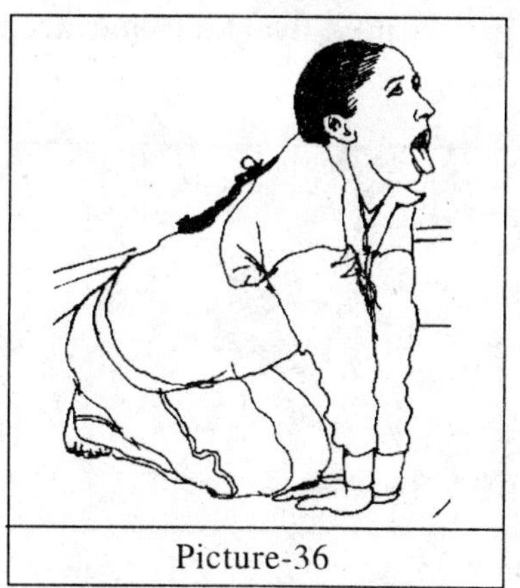
Picture-36

- Tilt the head backward, open the mouth and stretch the tongue outside the mouth as maximum as possible.
- Keep the eyes open widely, gazing the eyebrow centre and while exhaling produce the sound AA. AA. AA....AA from the voice box.

Vajrasana

- Sit back on the heels, keeping them apart and well tucked in under the buttocks.
- Keep the head, shoulders and buttocks in a straight line.

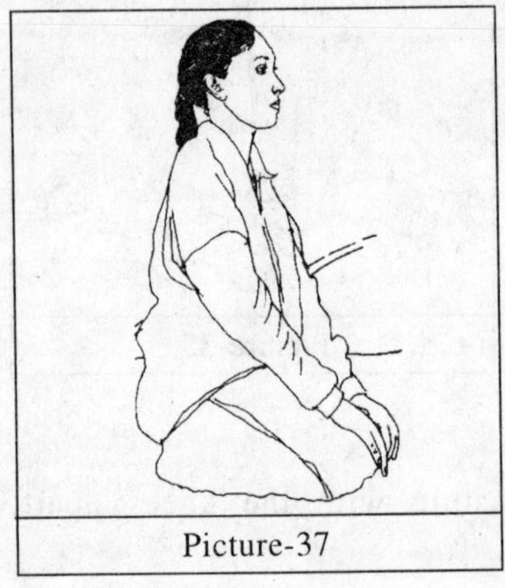
Picture-37

- The hands should rest on respective thighs, with palms facing down on the top of thighs.
- Keep the breathing normal and calm.
- It may be practised for maximum possible duration, especially straight after meals for at least 5-10 minutes.

Supta Vajrasana

- Sit in Vajrasana.
- Raise the knees and thighs a little off the floor; recline back on the floor; take two long and deep breaths.

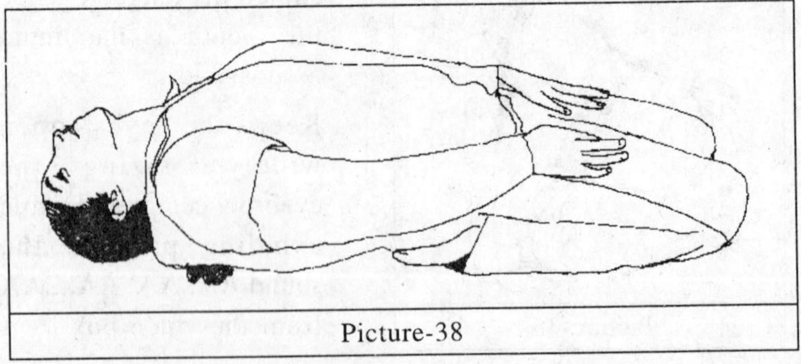
Picture-38

- Stretch the neck back so that the crown of the head rests on the floor; arch the chest and trunk up.
- Keep the hands on thighs and ensure that thighs are now touching the ground.
- Relax the body while keeping the eyes closed.
- Breathing should remain slow, deep and calm.

Ushtrasana

- Kneel on the floor, keeping the thighs and feet a little apart, toes pointing back and resting on the floor.
- Rest the palms on the hips; stretch the thighs; curve the spine back and extend the ribs.
- Now exhale, place the right palm on the right heel and left palm over the left heel.
- Press the feet with palms, throw the head and neck backward.
- Keep the body weight on the arms.
- Remain in this position for about 30 seconds while keeping the breath normal.
- Release the hands one by one and return to kneeling position and then sit on the floor and relax.

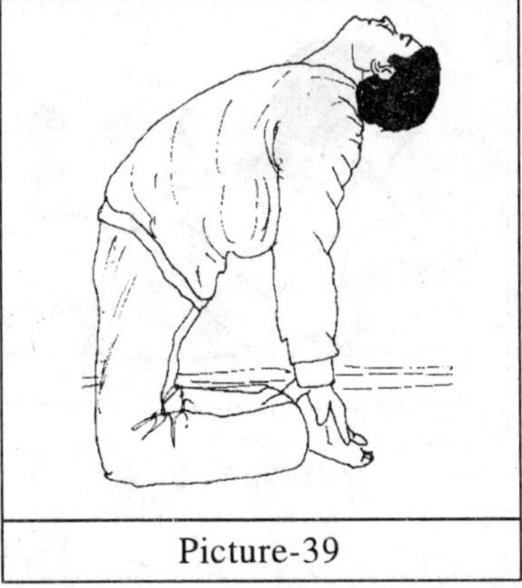

Picture-39

Bhujangasana

- Lie down in prone position, with legs straight and feet extended and together.
- Keep the forehead pressed to the ground.
- Completely relax the body in this posture.
- Then breathe in, press the head back and slowly raise the head and shoulders off the ground by bending the neck and back muscles.
- Straighten the arms gradually but without any unusual pressure on them: look at sky; hold the breath.
- Keep the navel very close to the ground.
- Try to maintain the posture as long as you can.
- Exhale and slowly return to the normal position; the forhead and chin touching the ground; and relax.
- Repeat it 2-3 times.

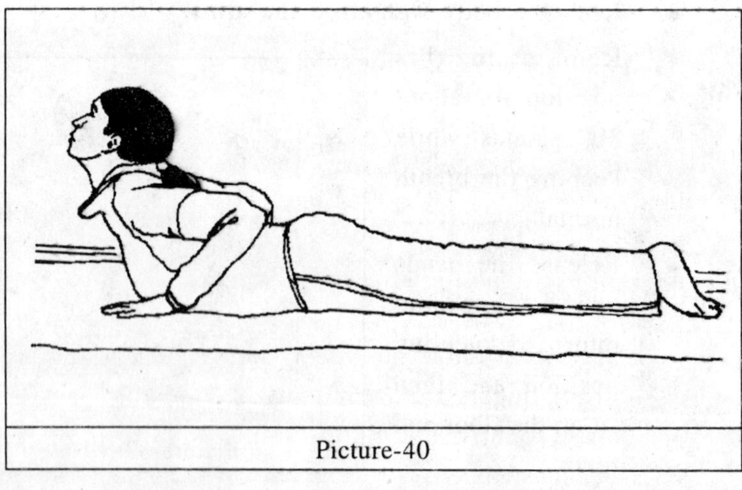

Picture-40

Shalabhasana

- Lie face downwards on the floor, hands and legs stretched, legs together, arms by sides, hands tightly clenched.
- Stretch the neck out but the chin on the floor and not the face.
- Inhale and raise both the legs together as high as possible without any bend at the knee.
- Hold the position for maximum duration, exhale and lower the legs slowly.

Repeat the process 2-3 times.

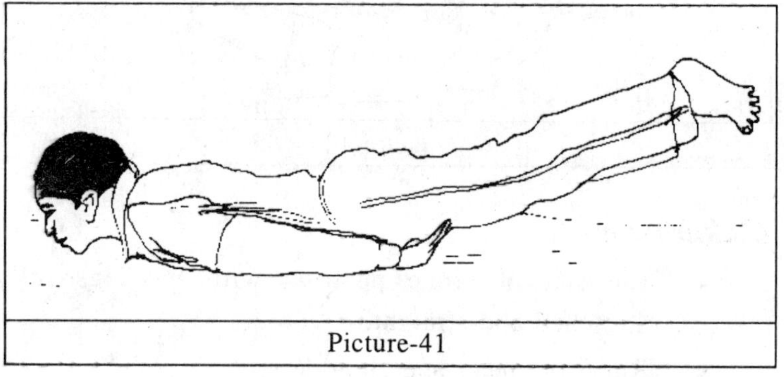

Picture-41

Dhanurasana

- Assume the prone posture face down on the floor, feet together and legs stretched, hands by sides.
- Inhale.
- Raise your chin, and grasp your ankles by putting all the fingers and thumb over ankle bone; part the knees slightly, but big toes and inside lines of the feet must touch.

- Push the feet back and up in one movement and bring the head, chest and thighs as high as possible.
- Keep the arms straight.
- Hold the position for as long as you feel comfortable.
- Exhale and come back in the basic prone posture and relax.

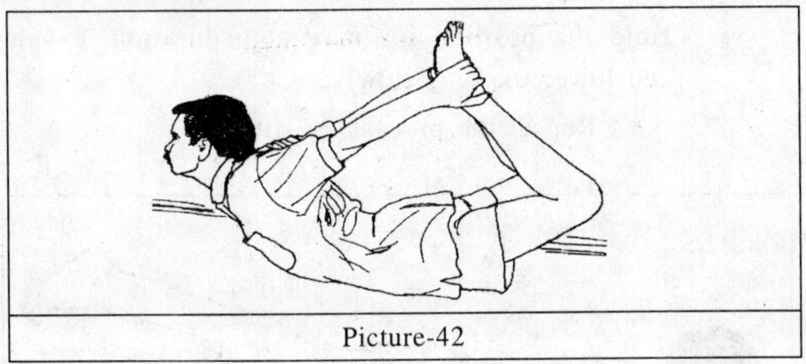

Picture-42

Makarasana

- Lie flat in prone position with the legs fully stretched and straight.
- Raise the head and shoulders.

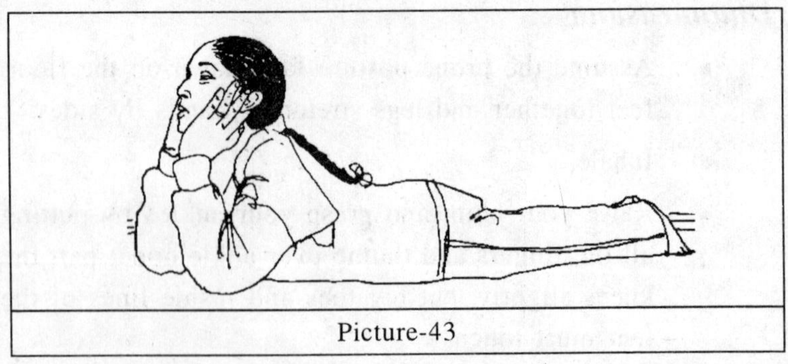

Picture-43

- Fold the hands, place the elbow on the floor, and hold the face and chin in the palms.
- Close the eyes and relax the whole body.

Uttan Padasana

- Lie down in supine position, legs stretched and feet together, hands comfortably at sides.
- While inhaling lift the legs, both together.
- Stop at 30^0 angle for a few seconds and bring back the legs on the ground, while exhaling.
- Again inhale and lift the legs up to 60^0; stop there and come back; exhale.
- Keep the legs straight while lifting upward and coming back to the ground.
- It you find this too strenuous, try with one leg at a time, using slow movement and repeating the movement at least twice on each side.

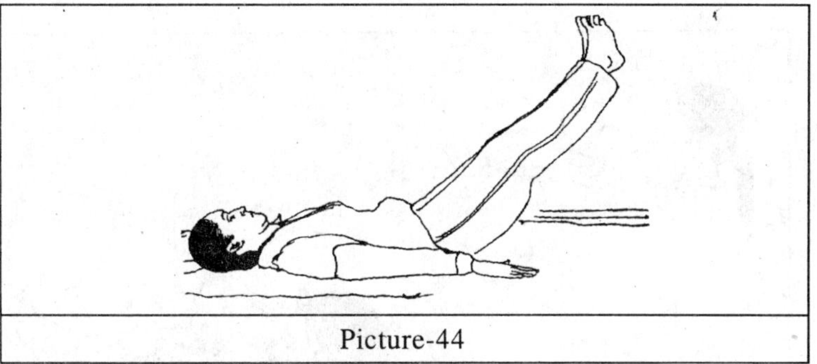

Picture-44

Pawan Muktasana

- Lie down in supine position, legs fully stretched and hands by sides.

- Lift the legs a little off the ground and give them a twist towards right side from the hips, while inhaling.
- Bring them back in straight line with the body, while exhaling.
- While inhaling fold the legs from knees and bring them towards head and trunk.
- Encircle both the knees by hands, lift the head and neck off the ground and place the nose between the knees, while inhaling.
- Hold the position for 10-15 seconds.
- Exhale and bring back the head and neck on the ground.
- Release the hands and stretch the legs and bring both of them on the ground.
- Repeat the process on the left side also.
- Do this exercise 2-3 times.

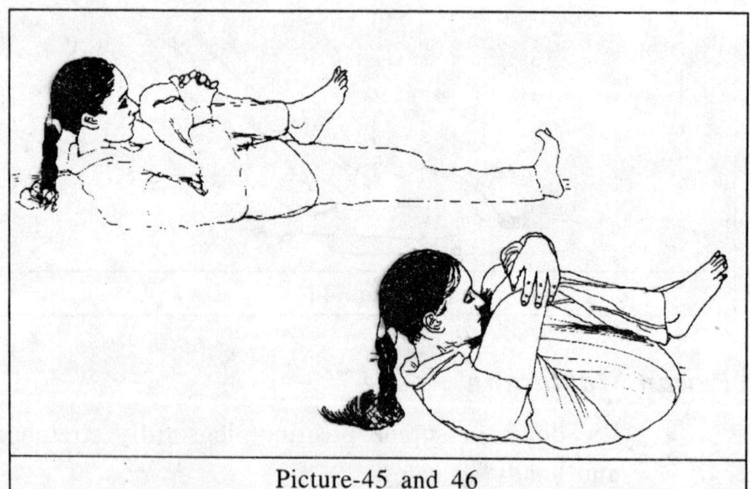

Picture-45 and 46

Halasana

- Lie down on the floor in a supine position with the arms at the sides and feet together.
- Breathe in and lift both the legs together in a vertical position.
- Breathe out and bend the trunk upward and carry the legs over the head, lower them till both the toes touch the floor at the back.
- Do not take the help of arms at all and always keep the legs straight and the knees stiff.
- Keep the arms flat on the floor, hands locked together.
- Maintain the posture as long as you can comfortably.
- Slowly return to the floor, rolling the body down from the shoulders, down the mid-back and finally the lower back till you are once again lying with back supine on the floor.
- The head must be firm on the floor while coming back to the basal position.

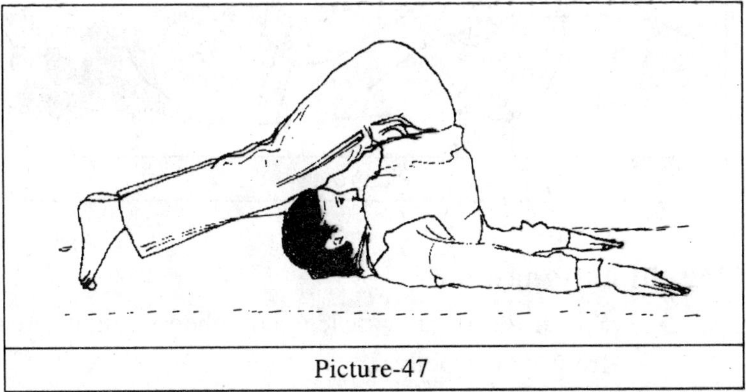

Picture-47

Matsyasana

- Assume a sitting position with the legs folded in the lotus pose.
- Arch and bend back, supporting the body on both the elbows and let the crown of head touch the ground; also arch the chest as high as possible.
- Hold the toes and rest the elbows on the floor.
- In the advanced form of Matsyasana the body rests on the firm base formed by the folded legs and on the head, without any support of elbows.
- Breathe deeply and stay in this position for as long as possible.
- Then release the neck and let the head rest on the floor; straighten legs; relax the hands and elbows; and relax finally.

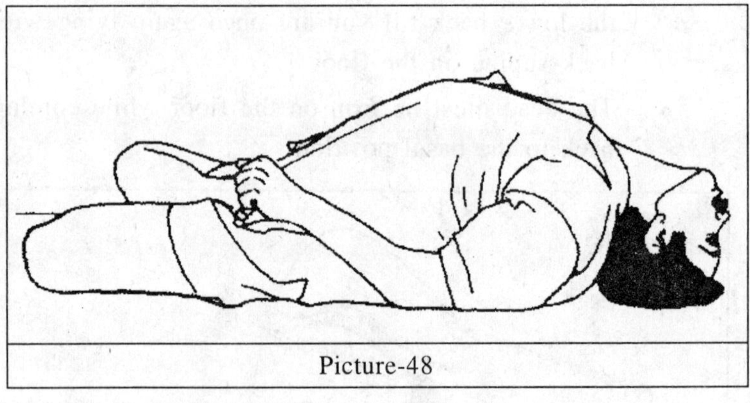

Picture-48

Paschimottanasana

- Sit on the floor with legs stretched straight out in front of the body.

- Exhale and bend forward to catch the big toes with the fingers and thumb.
- Keep the knees stiff and lower the elbows downwards on either side of the knees.
- Hold the position for a few seconds.
- Breathe in and pull the trunk lower, toward the legs, slowly and very gently, without any excessive strain.
- Try to touch the knees with your forehead to complete the pose.
- Remain in the pose as long as you can easily and comfortably and then return to the basal sitting position.
- Relax and repeat the exercise 2-3 times.

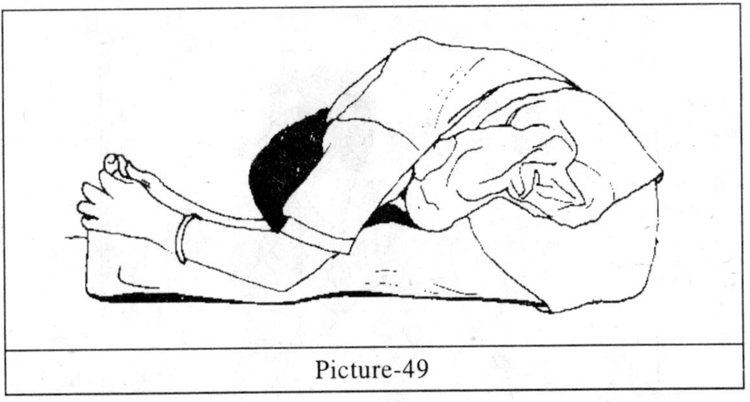

Picture-49

Ardha Matsyendrasana

- Sit on the floor with the legs extended in front, and feet together.

- Double up the right leg and place the foot against the outside surface of the left knee with the ankle touching that knee.
- Keep the right foot flat on the ground, parallel.
- Now place the left arm against the knee of the bent right leg, the armpit resting on the knee.
- Bring the left hand up to the extended left leg and try to touch the shin or if possible the right foot.
- Turn the body to right, placing the right arm behind the back.
- Give easily possible twist to the back and neck without excessive strain.
- Remain in the final pose for a few seconds and then slowly return to the starting position.
- Repeat the exercise by changing the leg to the other side.

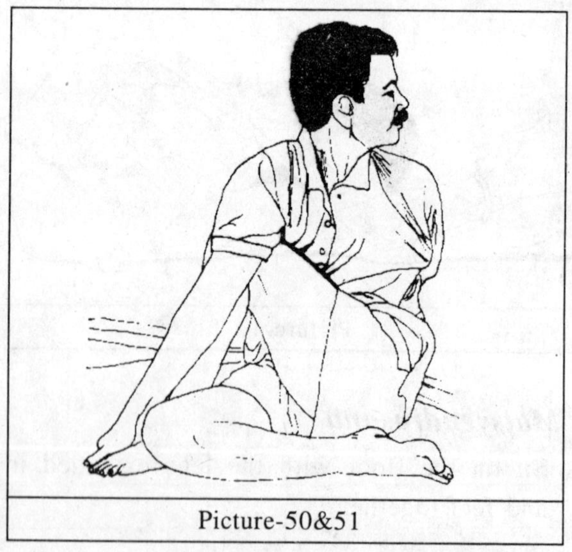

Picture-50&51

Naukasana

- Lie flat in supine position.
- Keep the legs extended in front, arms straight at the sides, palms facing down.
- While inhaling lift the legs, arms, trunk and head.
- Raise the head and feet not more than a foot (30 cm).
- The arms should be raised in the level of toes.
- Remain in this position as long as you can comfortably.
- Return to starting position while exhaling.
- Relax the whole body.
- Repeat the exercise for 4-5 times.

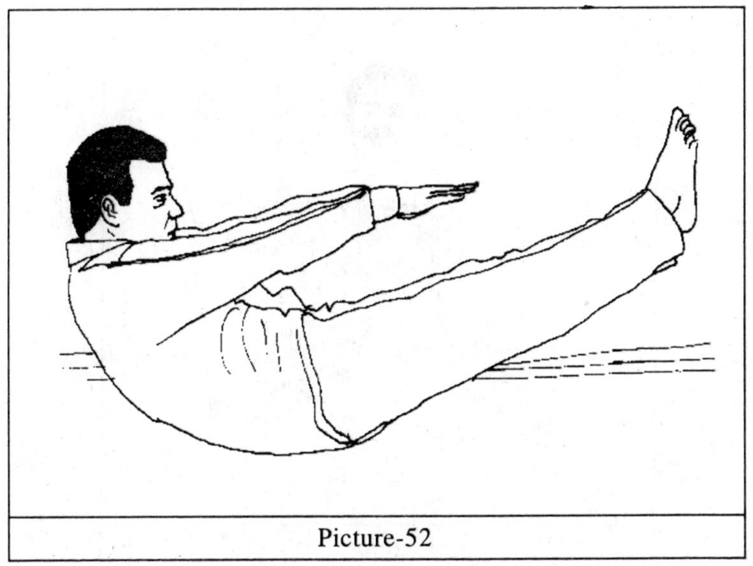

Picture-52

Siddhasana

- Assume a sitting posture with legs straight in front of the body.
- Bend the right leg from the knee and draw the heel close to the perineum; the leg from the knee to the heel must lie flat along the floor.
- Now bend the left leg at the knee and place it by foot on top of the right calf.
- The legs should be locked with the knees on the ground, and right and left heel should remain very close to each other.
- Stretch the arms out and the back of hands on the knees, palms upward.
- Make the spine straight, erect and steady, join the thumbs and forefingers together to make a circle and extend other fingers straight out.

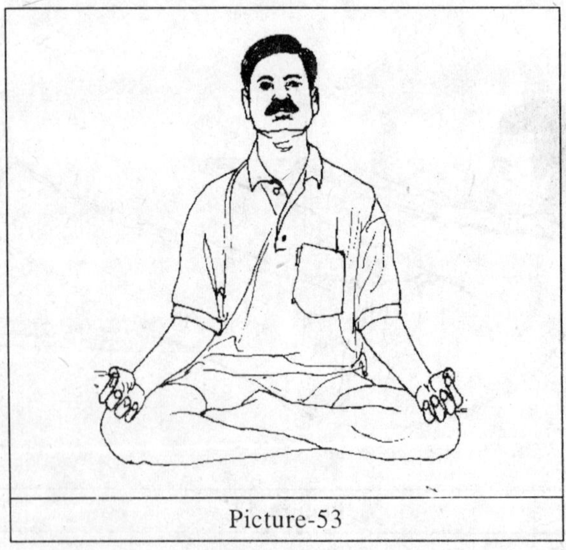

Picture-53

Sarvangasana

- Lie down in a supine position, with legs and arms extended straight; palms facing downward on the ground.
- Take a deep breath and lift both the legs back to vertical position, till they are at right angle to the body.
- Pause and exhale.
- Inhale and swing legs, buttocks and lower back off the floor, supporting the back with hands high up just under the shoulders and rising the body till it is straight and perpendicular to the chin, which is pressed tightly into the sternum.
- In case of difficulty in the begining to attain this position, you may bend the knees and fold the legs against the thighs before lifting them up.
- Hold the breath inside while assuming and returning from this exercise and keep the rhythmic breathing while in raised posture.

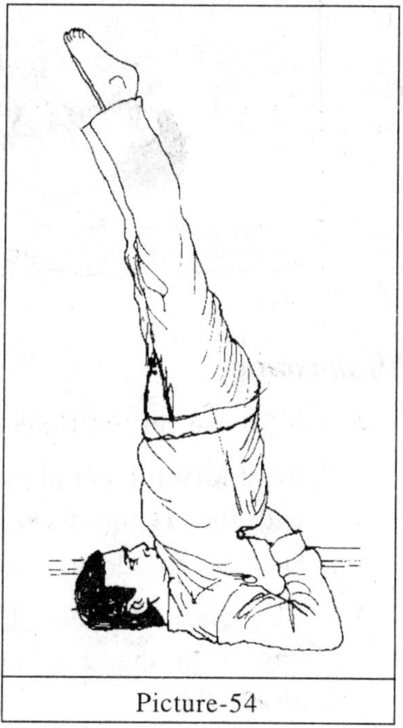

Picture-54

Vipareet Karni

- The basic technique for this exercise is the same as for Sarvangasana, with the difference that the chin is not pressed into the sternum in the final posture. The trunk should not be raised at right angle, instead it should be held at 45 degrees only.

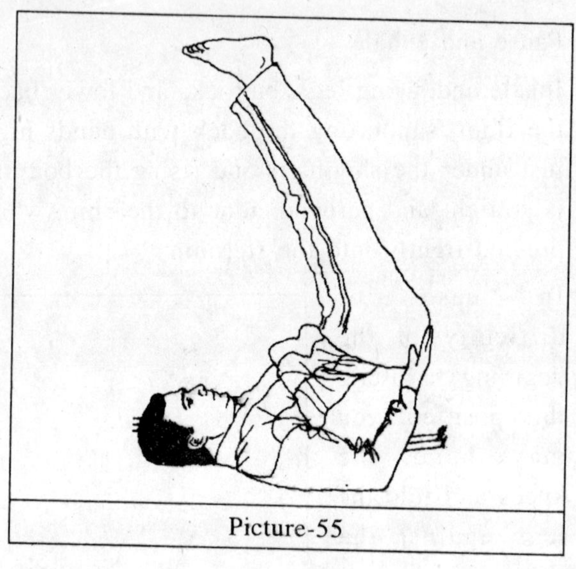

Picture-55

Shirshasana

- Sit down on the floor in Vajrasana.
- Bend forward and place the forearms on the ground with fingers interlocked and the elbows in front of knees at an adequate distance (Stage-I).
- Now place the head in the triangle of interlocked fingers in the way so that it touches the floor (Stage-II).

- Now walk up, straightening the knees until the back is perpendicular to the floor (Stage-III).
- Take a deep inhalation and lift the knees by pulling in close to the body; the back is straight and balanced, the toes pointing upward (Stage-IV); lean slightly back to maintain the balance.
- After coming in steady position at stage no. IV, raise the legs slowly and extend them up straight until the whole body comes in a vertical line, totally balanced on head and elbows.
- Breathe slowly and deeply and hold the position up to comfortable length of time without any excessive strain.
- To come back to the original kneeling position first bend the knees, then the body at the hips and finally lower the legs till the feet are touching the floor.
- In the beginning you may take support of a wall for completely raising the legs.

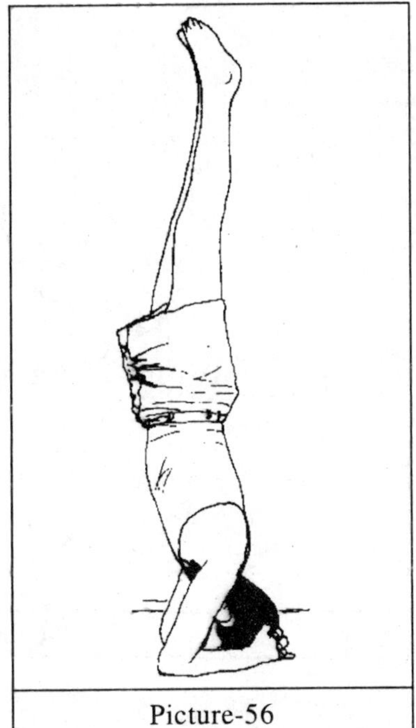

Picture-56

Shavasana

- Lie flat in a supine position.
- Keep legs extended and arms beside and in the line of the body, palms facing sky.
- Keep the feet apart at 1 foot (30 cm) distance.
- Close the eyes.
- Do not move any part of the body at all.
- Relax the body.
- Let the breath become long, deep, calm and rhythmic.
- Be aware of each inhalation and exhalation.
- Concentrate your mind on breath only.

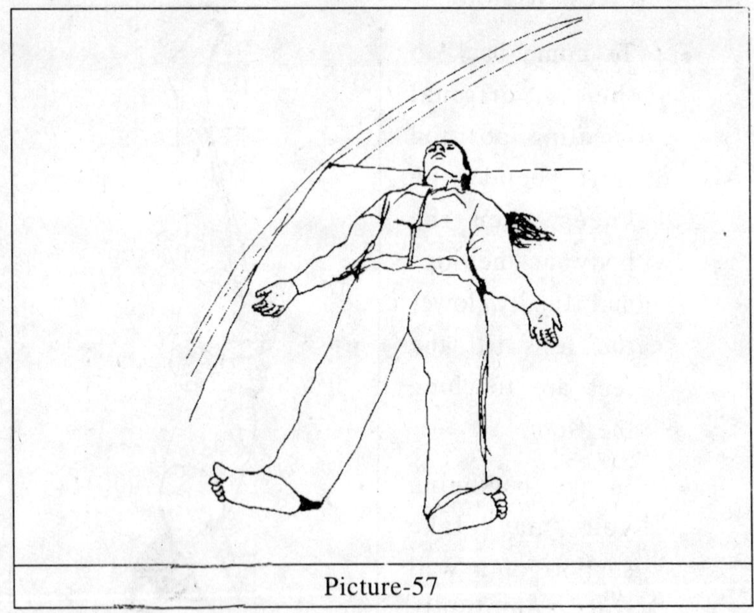

Picture-57

MUDRA AND BANDH

- Maha mudra 126
- Gyan mudra 127
- Sambhavi mudra 128
- Tadagi mudra 128
- Kaki mudra 129
- Bhujangini mudra 129
- Ashwini mudra 130
- Yoni mudra 131
- Akashi mudra 131
- Jalandhar bandh 132
- Uddiyan bandh 133
- Mool bandh 134

Mudra and Bandh

In the sacred ancient yoga texts it has been mentioned that mudras are more powerful than asanas and pranayama as they are instrumental in awakening the hidden serpent power in human being — the **Kundalini shakti**. In *Gherand Samhita,* the most authentic yoga text, 25 odd mudras are explained. A mudra is a specific position representing specific state of psyche. Sometimes mudras are being used to regulate several involuntary physiological and biochemical activities. Mudras have been proved to help in developing self awareness about the flow of vital energy in the subtle body. Mudras also enhance spiritual orientation and promote the process of **self healing** as well as **psychic healing**.

Bandhs are another small group of yogic techniques which enable the practitioner to control his organs at his will. As it is self-explanatory, **Bandh** means **'to hold or tighten'**. Contracting and tightening different body parts and organs give a regular massage to them, coordinate the functions of central nervous system (CNS), peripheral nervous system (PNS) and autonomic nervous system (ANS), along with improving the blood circulation at the places where blood is stagnant. Although bandhs are performed physically and locally, their effect is deep and on the whole body.

Maha Mudra

- Assume a sitting posture.
- Place the left heel under the arms and right leg extended forward.
- Lean forward and catch hold of the toes with both hands.

- First inhale and then exhale deeply and hold the breath outside.
- Contract the throat and gaze in the centre between the eyebrows.
- Repeat the process with the other leg also.

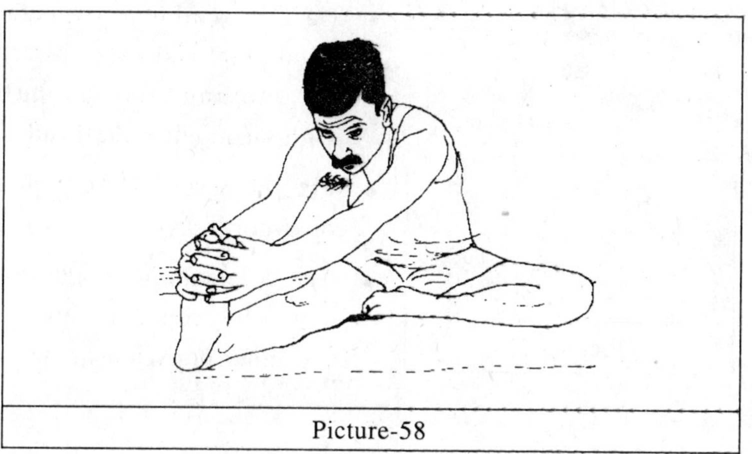

Picture-58

Gyan Mudra

- Sit in a meditative asana, say Padmasana or Sukhasana.
- Place the straightened hand on the knees with palm facing the sky; fold both the index fingers and join it with respective thumbs; keep the other three fingers straight.

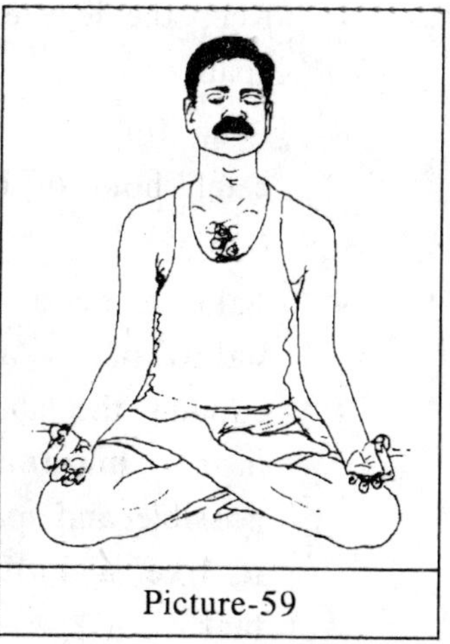

Picture-59

Sambhavi Mudra

- Assume a meditative asana posture.

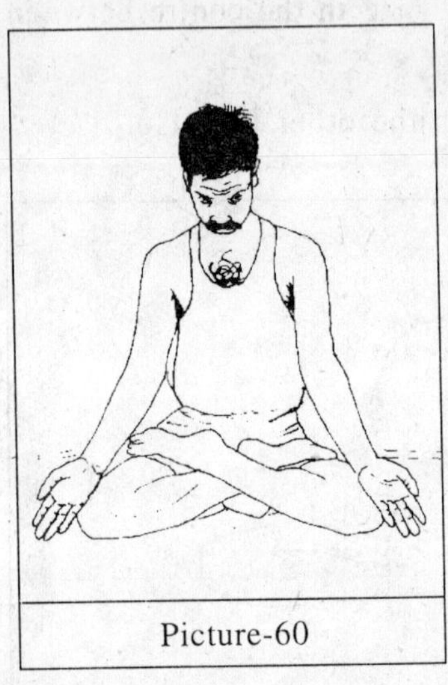
Picture-60

- Keep the spine straight and place the straightened hands on the knees.
- Gaze forward at a particular fixed point and look upward by moving the eyeball without moving the head.
- Fix the gaze at the centre of eyebrows.
- Try to remain in thoughtless state, by concentrating on the inner consciousness.

Tadagi Mudra

- Assume a sitting posture.
- Keep the legs extended forward and feet slightly apart.
- Lean forward and catch hold of big toes.
- Take a deep inhalation, and expand the abdomen maximum possible and make it like a hollow tank.

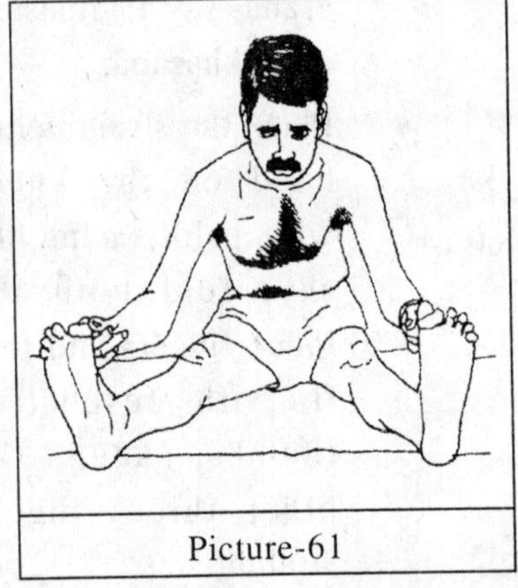
Picture-61

- Hold the breath inside for the maximum length of time.
- Then exhale and relax without leaving the toes.
- Now inhale and exhale repeatedly.
- Inhale and repeat the process 5-6 times.

Kaki Mudra

- Adopt a sitting meditative posture.
- Make a narrow cannal with the help of lips, in the shape of the beak of a crow.
- Concentrate on the tip of nose.
- Inhale slowly and deeply through mouth and then close the lips.
- Then exhale through the nose.
- Repeat the process several times.

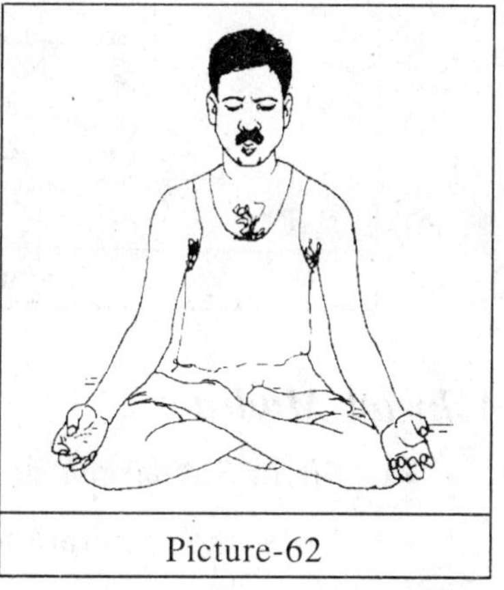

Picture-62

Bhujangini Mudra

- Sit in comfortably, assuming a meditative pose.
- Relax the body.
- Extrude the mouth a little forward and try to drink the air with the gullet into the stomach not the lungs, as if you are drinking water.
- Expand the stomach as much as possible.

- Retain the air inside for a short duration and then expel it noisily through the mouth.
- Repeat the process several times.

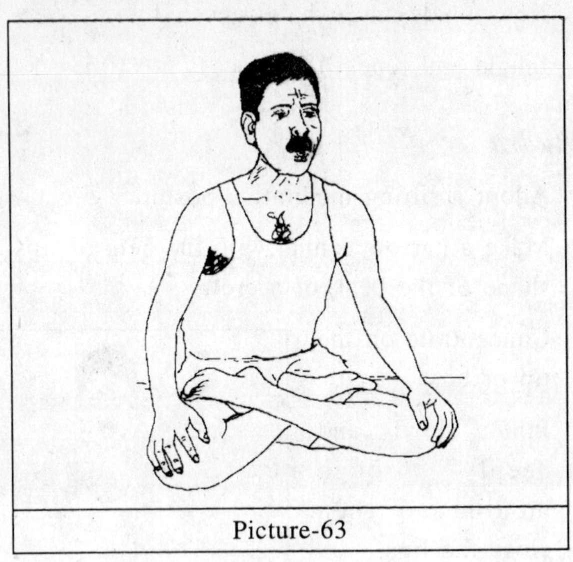

Picture-63

Ashwini Mudra

- Sit in Sukhasana or Padmasana.
- Make the respiration regular and rhythmic.
- Close the eyes and relax the body.
- Contract and expand the sphincter muscles of the anus repeatedly.
- Inhale and hold the breath while contracting the sphincter muscles, and while expanding exhale slowly.
- Do not exert any excessive strain and repeat the process several times.

Yoni Mudra

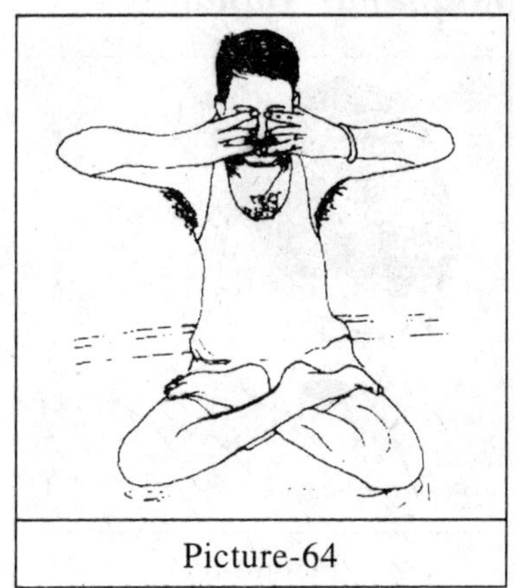
Picture-64

- Assume a sitting meditative posture.
- Inhale slowly and deeply and retain the breath inside.
- Close the eyes with index fingers, ears with the thumbs and nostrils with the middle fingers, while placing the ring and little fingers over the mouth.
- Concentrate on internal manifestation of sound echo.
- Open the nostrils only and exhale.
- Again inhale and close the nostrils.
- Repeat the exercise several times for the maximum length of time available.

Akashi Mudra

- Adopt a sitting meditative posture.
- Fold the tongue in backward direction as is being done in Khechari mudra.
- Now perform Ujjayi pranayama along with Sambhavi mudra.
- At the same time tilt the head a little backward.
- Breath should be slow and deep.
- Repeat the process a few times.

Jalandhar Bandh

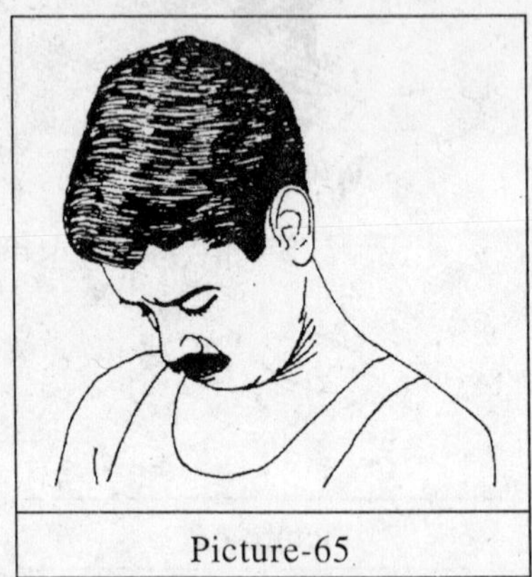
Picture-65

- Assume a sitting posture, preferably Padmasana or Sukhasana.
- Both the knees should firmly touch the ground.
- Place the palms of straightened hands on the knees.
- Close the eyes and relax the body.
- Take a deep inhalation, hold the breath inside and bend the head forward — downward. Now press the chin tightly into the sternum.
- Pull the shoulders up and bend them forward into a rounded shape, while keeping the hand straight and palms firm on the knees.
- Continue to remain in this pose as long as you can.
- Now relax the shoulders and arms, slowly raise the head and exhale.
- Repeat the procedure after the normal breathing is achieved.
- This exercise can also be performed in standing position.

Uddiyana Bandh

- Sit in a comfortable meditative pose.
- Both the knees should rest on the ground firmly, and palms over them.

- Close the eyes and relax the whole body.
- Exhale completely and hold the breath outside.
- Perform Jalandhar bandh.
- Now suck in the abdomen, raise the diaphragm and expand the chest; abdominal wall is now flattened against the spine and a hollow cavity is formed.
- When you can no longer hold the breath, relax the muscles and allow the air to enter the lungs in a long slow inhalation and return to basic relaxing position.
- Breath normally and then repeat the whole procedure.

This exercise can be practised in the standing position too.

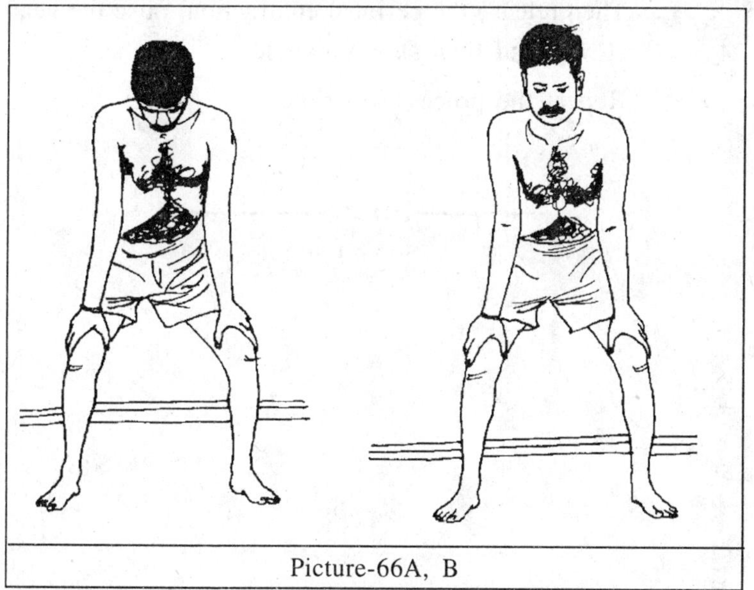

Picture-66A, B

Mool Bandh

This exercise may be performed in standing, sitting, or lying position, but the best posture is Siddhasana or Mool bandh asana, because in this posture heel is being pressed into the perineum and thereby automatically it helps in the performance.

- Sit in Siddhasana with knees touching the ground and palms on the knees.
- Take a deep inhalation, hold the breath inside and perform Jalandhar bandh.
- Now try to contract the ring of muscles around the anus tightly and up, thereby causing the whole pelvic region to contract.
- Retain the posture for the easily possible maximum length of time along with breath retention.
- Then release the perineal contraction, raise the head slowly and then slowly exhale.
- Repeat the process 4-5 times.

———:::::::::———

KAYOTSARGA

- Progressive relaxation 137
- Applied relaxation programme 137
- Instant relaxation technique (IRT), quick relaxation technique (QRT) and deep relaxation technique (DRT) 139
- Kayotsarga 139

Kayotsarga *(Relaxation)*

Tense, overwrought, nervous and anxious, modern man is caught up in the hellish grind which drives him inexorably into stress, because his constant state of anxiety prevents him from facing up to the relentless demand of modern life which, behind an amiable and comfortable exterior, conceals an inhuman machine and an unrelenting struggle for existence. It is really surprising, then, that millions of civilized beings live with depressing feeling that they are 'out of step', overlaid by apparently impossible tasks with which they cannot possibly cope, and from which they can never escape. Tranquilizers, the 'happy' pills of modern chemistry, do bring an apparent respite, but in long run the remedy is worse than the disease, since it does no more than dampen the roots of this anxiety and nervousness without eradicating them. But there are two sorts of remedies, both preventive and curative — controlled breathing and relaxation; the latter is the most direct antidote.

When we point out that the relaxation must be learnt, we may seem to be pointing to some far-off goal, and many people come to yoga for instant help with immediate problems. We live at a faster pace than the average oriental, and our forebearers were probably living at a faster pace than the founders of yoga thousands of years ago. But the paths of yoga are such that immediate benefit can be gained from the very start of every new discipline, from the first yoga breath we draw and the first asana we attempt, and from our basic training in relaxation. We do not have to reach a state of perfection to start to enjoy results. It benefits us more to start to relax in the proper yoga fashion than to become mechanically adept in any other type of relaxation exercise ever devised. This is because yoga relaxation is complete, relaxing not only muscles but also internal organs, glandular system, lungs, heart, nervous system and **mind** as well. A few specific relaxation techniques are being described here.

Progressive Relaxation

Edmund Jacobson, a Chicago physician, has described the new technique of relaxation known as **progressive relaxation**. According to Dr Jacobson it requires no imagination, will power or suggestion and it is based on the promise that the body responds to anxiety — provoking thoughts and events with muscle tension. This physiological tension, in turn, increases the subjective experience of anxiety. Deep muscle relaxation reduces physiological tension and is incompatible with anxiety.

Excellent results were obtained in the treatment of muscular tension, anxiety, insomnia, depression, fatigue, irritable bowel, muscle spasm, neck and back pain, hypertension etc., in the short duration of only 2 weeks, obseving two sessions of 15 min. every day regularly without any break.

Applied Relaxation Programme

The technique of **applied relaxation** was developed by a Swedish physician L. G. Ost in 1988. While working with phobic patients, who needed rapid and reliable methods to cut through the anxiety that struck when they encountered phobic situations, he observed that this technique achieved high rates of success, also that it could be helpful in a variety of life situations from daily fights and frustrations to chronic insomnia.

Applied relaxation training progresses in the following six stages:

Progressive relaxation: It helps in recognising the difference between tension and relaxation in each major group of muscles.

Release-only relaxation: It cuts out the first step in progressive muscle relaxation — the tensing step. That means one can cut the time down by more than half to achieve deep relaxation in each muscle group.

Cue-controlled relaxation: It reduces the time needed to relax even further, down to 2-3 minutes. In this stage one has to focus on the **breathing**, and to condition himself to relax exactly when desired. Such instruction helps in building an association between a cue and true muscle relaxation.

Differential relaxation: At this stage the practitioner is able to sit down in a chair at any point of time during the day and achieve deep relaxation in a few minutes. This advance stage helps the practitioner relax while busy in his daily activities. Differential relaxation helps isolate the specific muscles needed for the activity done at the time of relaxation, and allow the rest of the body to relax. It lets him do so in a variety of settings.

Rapid relaxation: This cuts down further the time needed to relax to only 30 seconds. Being able to relax that quickly can mean real relief during stressful life situations. It is good and extremely useful to practice rapid relaxation many times a day as one has to move through different activities and states of mind.

Applied relaxation: The final stage of applied relaxation training involves relaxing quickly in the face of anxiety-provoking situations. At this stage the performer is in full command to cut down the anxiety reactions before they build up.

Instant Relaxation Technique (IRT), Quick Relaxation Technique (QRT) and Deep Relaxation Technique (DRT)

These three relaxation techniques were developed by Vivekananda Kendra Yoga Research Foundation, Bangalore. These are quite effective and easy-to-perform relaxation techniques. IRT can be practised after every individual exercise for a short duration. QRT or DRT can be performed after the asanas or independently between the daily routine to provide adequate and real rest to the body systems.

Kayotsarga

Kayotsarga is the total relaxation with self awareness. The existence of mental stress as a part of modern living has been universally accepted. Repeated stressful situations not only affect our psychological status negatively but also undermine our physical health. In the so-called modern age, the age of overactivity and daily hassel, conscious relaxation is a panacea for many maladies and problems, because such working culture and undue restlessness produce mental distress and psychosomatic disorders. The only safe remedy is conscious relaxation and deliberate suspension of all bodily movements.

Kayotsarga literally means abandonment of the body coupled with high degree of conscious awareness. In practice, it is conscious suspension of all gross movements of the body, resulting in relaxation of the skeletal muscles and drastic reduction in metabolic activities. This physical condition results in relieving mental tension and is an essential precondition of meditational practice, although it may be practised independently for the desired duration. If one learns and practises systematic relaxation every day, one would remain relaxed, calm and unperturbed in any situation. Physically, it is more restful than sleep, and is the direct antidote to psychosomatic maladies resulting from tension. Spiritually, in this process the lifeless body is cast off, whereas the consciousness soars upward, freed from and outside its material shell. Kayotsarga is not only total relaxation, but also actual perception of the *self,* quite apart from the material *non- self.* (— Acharya Mahaprgya and Muni Mahendra Kumar)

For proper appraisal of relaxation we must know the muscular functions. The muscle may be compared to an electromagnet and the nerve that stimulates it to action to an electric wire which connects it to the brain. During sleep, very poor current circulates in the nerves, and the muscles are almost demagnetised, whereas in rest period a weak current flows through nerves, barely magnetising the muscles, which are in a quiescent state. In another peculiar state, the state of hypertension, electromagnets are overmagnetised by very strong current, leaving various muscle groups in the state of shockful contraction and expansion. By conscious voluntary efforts it is well possible to switch off the electrical current inflow to those muscles, which ultimately results in the proved relaxation.

However, true relaxation can ever be acquired by force. It is basically an exercise of the mastery of conscious will over the body by the technique of autosuggestion. In our heritage of ancient medical texts it is well elaborated that apart from nature healing, diet, medicinal herbs, bone setting, minor surgery etc., there was a concept of faith-healing, in which the patients were treated through suggestions.

The technique of autosuggestion (and suggestion) is the most ancient psychotherapy known to mankind. People of every culture and belief have not only explored the higher states of consciousness by taking the use of this technique, but also they used it to heal the sick through relaxation and suggestion. In the recent days the technique has gained the acceptance by both British Medical Association and American Medical Association.

Autosuggestion is the basic principle of the technique of kayotsarga. Each part of the body is relaxed, in turn by coaxing autosuggestion.

Technique of kayotsarga:

- Sit in comfortable meditational posture (in Padmasana or Sukhasana).
- Keep the eyes closed softly.
- Inhale deeply and silently for about 4 to 5 seconds, concentrating your attention on cranium (head), and pressing your lips together exhale slowly without interruption.
- Produce the sound like the buzzing of a bee.
- This may last for about 8 -10 seconds.
- Inhale deeply again and repeat the performance nine times.
- Then either maintain the same posture or lie down in supine pose; the legs fully stretched and foot a little apart. Keep the hands also stretched and in the sides with palms facing upward.
- Maintain the posture, keeping the neck, spine, buttocks and both the heels in touch with the floor.

- Relax all the muscles of your body and let the body become limp.
- Concentrate your mind on each part of the body, one by one. Allow each part to relax by the process of autosuggestion and feel that it has become relaxed.
- Starting with the big toe of the right foot, allow your mind to spread throughout the toe; suggest to the muscles and nerves to relax; experience the resulting relaxation and pass on the other parts of the right leg — toes, sole, heel, ankle, upper part of the foot, calf muscle, knees, thighs and buttocks. In the same way, relax the left leg up to the hip joint.
- Now relax the trunk from hip joint to the neck, passing through every part one by one.
- Then relax both limbs — fingers, thumbs, palms, wrist, lower arms, elbow and upper arms.
- Then relax both the shoulders and upper neck portion.
- Finally relax the head and adjoining parts — throat, chin, jaws, lips, tongue, cheeks, nose, eyes, ears, forehead and scalp.
- Then experience that the whole body is completely relaxed and is full of freshness.
- Retain the relaxed condition as desired.

——— :::::::: ———

PRANAYAMA

- Ujjayai 148
- Suryabhedi 149
- Nadi shodhan 150
- Bhastrika 150
- Sheetali 152
- Sheetkari 153
- Bhramari 154
- Anulom vilom 154

Pranayama

We are aware of vital importance of breath, without which we cannot survive, but a few of us are willing to face a fact that most of us know, that our breathing is usually inadequate for the body's needs, that we breath shallowly and lazily, so that the blood is seldom, if ever, sufficiently oxygenated.

The implications of this inadequate breathing style are more far-reaching than is generally supposed. Many of the vague symptoms of poor health have their root cause in the fact that when blood is insufficiently oxygenated, circulation is slow, and not only are various internal organs and glands and nerves insufficiently nourished, but also the excretory system itself does not function efficiently and the bodily waste products are not removed.

Lack of oxygen is a prime cause of tiredness, brain fatigue and headaches, but in actuality the effects are deeper and more far-reaching. Oxygen is considered the vital fuel of the body and one cannot run the body at full strength on insufficient fuel.

The question arises why do we breathe so badly? There are four main reasons of this inadequate breathing.

- First, purely from habit, which has engendered a kind of passive laziness of which we are unaware.
- Second, the cramped position we assume during our working.
- Third, our bodies tend to be so stiff that many have actual difficulty in expanding the thoracic cage, so that the position of the lungs, bounded by the ribs, is seldom swelled to its full capacity.

- Fourth, we restrict our breathing by tight and heavy clothes. All this creates the condition that we breathe in an estimated one-fifth of our normal oxygen requirement and use approximately one-third of our lung capacity.

There are three distinct types of breathing being generated and conducted in three distinct parts of the body, which are as follows:

Thoracic breathing: It involves the raising of the ribs by the dilation of thoracic cage, and takes a considerable amount of effort. It is seldom practised unless deep breathing exercises are undertaken.

Clavicular breathing: It is the process of breathing in which the breath is introduced into the top of lungs by raising of the shoulder girdle. It is shallow and insufficient, because it leaves the rest of the lung static.

Abdominal breathing: In this process the base of lungs is filled with air, aided by lowering of the diaphragm. It is also known as *diaphragmatic breathing*. Although it does not represent the whole of the total and correct breathing procedure, it is the most efficient of the three methods, though still inadequate.

In yoga, great stress is laid upon correct and total breathing, and upon breath control. This is called **Pranayama**, made up two Sanskrit words — Prana and Ayama. 'Prana' means breath, respiration, life, vitality, energy or strength. It also denotes certain vital breath flow of 'Prana Vayus'. 'Ayama' means to stretch, control, extension, expansion, regulation or restraint. Thus the wordly meaning of Pranayama is the prolongation of breath and its restraint.

Prana is the vital or etheric force, which is spread all over, and can be perceived in all living and non-living things. According to Upanishads, prana is the principal force of life and consciousness. It is equated with the Self (Atma). It is the breath of life of all individuals in the universe, and when they die their individual breath dissolves into the cosmic breath. Prana is often termed as air we breath but in fact it is not only air; Prana is more subtle than air and it can be defined as the energy essence that prevails within everything in the universe.

In the ancient texts Prana is divided into five types of vital energy, i.e. Prana vayus. They are Prana, Apana, Samana, Udana and Vyana. They are specific aspects of one vital cosmic force, the primaeval principle of existence of all beings.

Thus the Pranayama is the sequence of techniques that stimulate and increase the vital energy, ultimately bringing about perfect control over the flow of Prana within the body, by moving the respiratory organs intentionally, intensively and rhythmically.

Pranayama consists of the following four stages:

1. *Puraka:* Long, slow controlled and sustained subtle flow of inhalation.
2. *Kumbhaka:* Controlled suspension and retention of breath inside after inhalation.
3. *Rechaka:* Long, slow and controlled exhalation.
4. *Shunyaka:* Suspension of breath after exhalation.

In the first stage of Puraka the whole system is being stimulated. In the second stage of Kumbhaka vital energy is being distributed throughout the body. In the third stage of Rechaka vitiated air, full of carbon dioxide and other toxins, is thrown out. In the stage of Shunyaka the whole system revitalizes itself by taking a little rest and going ahead to the next cycle. The movement of the respiratory organs includes horizontal expansion, vertical ascension and circumferential extension of the lungs and rib cage. (For the detailed processes and step-by-step techniques of Pranayama the readers are requested to consult the B.K.S. Iyengar's *Light on Pranayama,* the most authentic, elaborative and well explanatory monograph on the subject.)

Thus the purpose of Pranayama is two-fold — **entire harmony** and **complete mental control**. Pranayama is performed to bring under control the fickle mind. It is said that the control of prana leads to that of the mind and causes equality of vision overall. It generates happiness and deters the sensual objects from arising in the mind. It also regulates the thoughts, desires and actions, gives poise and tremendous will power needed for self-mastery and self-healing power.

Many types of Pranayama exercises have been devised and evolved to meet the physical, mental, intellectual, spiritual and therapeutic requirements of the practitioners under much fluctuating conditions. Techniques of a few important Pranayama exercises are given here:

- Nadi shodhan pranayama
- Sheetali pranayama
- Sheetkari pranayama
- Bhramari pranayama

- Bhastrika pranayama
  - Ujjayai pranayama
  - Surya bhedi pranayama
- Anulom-vilom pranayama

Ujjayai

- Sit in Padmasana or Sukhasana.
- Perform the Khechari mudra.
- Contract the glottis in the throat and take a deep inhalation, feeling as if you are breathing through the throat only.
- Adopt the posture of Jalandhar bandh while holding the breath.
- Close the eyes and exhale completely.
- Take a slow, deep and steady breath through both the nostrils, with feeling of incoming air on the roof of palate.
- Hold the breath for a second or two, and observe Mool bandh (state of antar kumbhaka).
- Now exhale slowly and steadily, with the feeling of the outgoing air on the roof of the palate.
- Have a gap of few seconds before the next inhalation (state of bahya kumbhaka). This completes one cycle of Ujjayai prananyama.
- Repeat the process several times, keeping the eyes closed throughout.

Suryabhedi

- Assume a comfortable sitting posture like Padmasana or Siddhasana.
- Keep the spine and head erect and rigid, and place the hands on the knees.
- Close the eyes and relax the body.
- Fold the right hand from the elbow and place the right thumb on the right side of the nose, the ring and little fingers on the left side of the nose, middle and index fingers on the forehead.
- Close the left nostril with ring finger and inhale deeply through right nostril.
- Now close both the nostrils and observe Jalandhar and Mool bandh.
- Hold on to this position for the maximum possible duration.
- Now release the bandhs and exhale through left nostril, while keeping the right nostril closed.
- Repeat the process many times.

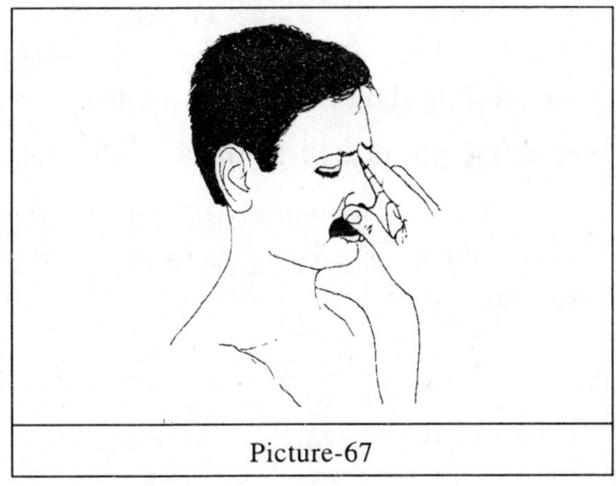

Picture-67

Nadi Shodhan

- Sit in meditative posture.
- Keep the spine erect and rigid and observe Jalandhar bandh.
- Stretch the arms and place them on the knees.
- Perform Gyan mudra by left hand.
- Fold the right hand from the elbow and place the right thumb on the right side and ring and little fingers on the left side of the nose, whereas middle and index fingers on the forehead.
- Block the left nostril by ring and little fingers and inhale slowly and deeply through right nostril.
- After full inhalation block the right nostril and exhale slowly and steadily through left nostril, emptying the lungs completely.
- After complete exhalation, now start inhaling through left nostril slowly and deeply, while keeping the right nostril closed.
- After complete inhalation block this nostril and start exhaling through the right nostril.
- Repeat the practice 10-15 times at a stretch.
- Always keep the thumb and finger position same and use them for closing and opening the nasal apertures.

Bhastrika

This pranayama is completed in two stages:

Stage-I

- Sit in Sukhasana or Padamasana position.
- Hold the head and back erect with eyes closed.
- Keep the left hand on the left knee and the index and middle fingers of right hand on forehead, while placing the little and ring fingers on one side and thumb on the other side of the nose.
- Close the right nostril and take fast, vigorous breath and exhale likewise fast and forcefully 15-20 times through left nostril, by expanding and contracting the abdomen.
- Take a deep inhalation, close both the nostrils and observe Jalandhar bandh. Hold the breath for as long as easily possible, release the bandh and then exhale slowly.
- Now close the left nostril, breathe likewise rapidly and forcefully through right nostril. Inhale deeply, observe Jalandhar bandh and hold the breath for a comfortable period and then slowly exhale.
- Repeat the whole process 2-3 times.

Stage-II

- Remain in the same sitting posture, but placing the hands on knees.
- Breathe vigorously and forcefully 15-20 times through both the nostrils.

- Take a deep inhalation, hold the breath and observe Jalandhar bandh and remain in the postion for some time.
- Then exhale slowly and repeat the process 3 to 5 times.

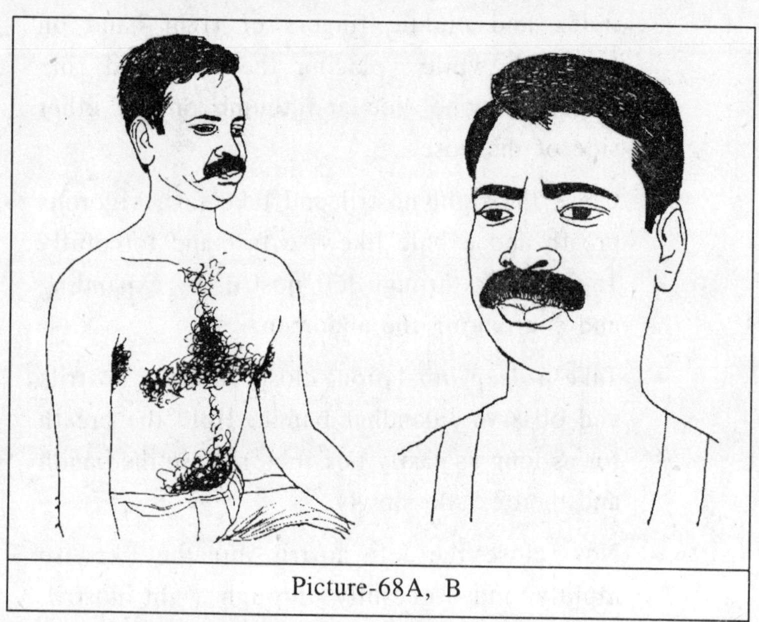

Picture-68A, B

Sheetali

- Adopt the posture of Padmasana or Sukhasana, keeping the back straight and hands in Gyan mudra.
- Open the mouth and give a circular shape to the lips like 'O' alphabet.
- Lift and curl up the tongue like a fresh leaf about to open or a narrow tube.
- Protrude the curled tongue outside the lips and inhale slowly and deeply through the narrow tube of folded tongue.

- After full inhalation, lower the head, and chin should rest in the notch between the collar bones.

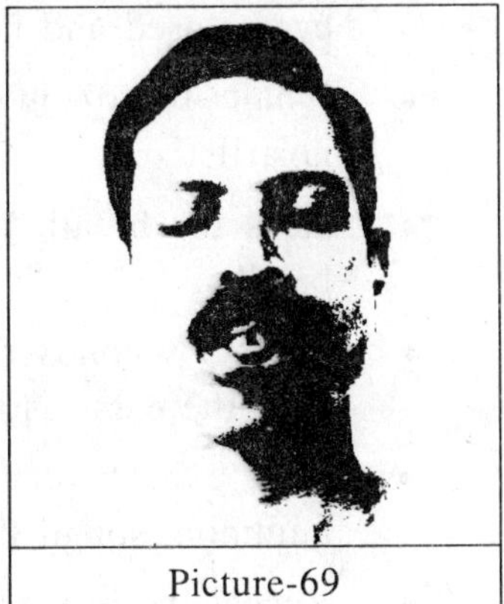

Picture-69

- Hold the breath for a few seconds, practising performing Jalandhar and Mool bandhs.
- After a few seconds release the lock of both the bandhs and exhale slowly through the nostrils.
- Repeat the exercise for 3 to 5 times.

Sheetkari

This is a simple variation of Sheetali pranayama.

- Here the tongue is folded to make a canal. Keep the lips slightly parted and only the tip of tongue protrudes between the teeth, keeping its shape flat as it is in usual state.

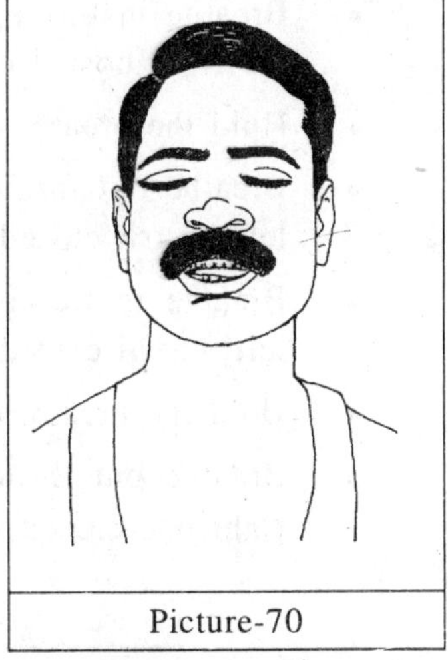

Picture-70

- Now inhale fully through the window of teeth and perform Jalandhar and Mool bandhs.
- After some time release the bandhs and exhale slowly through nose.

Bhramari

- Assume a sitting meditative asana posture, with eyes closed and head and spine erect.
- Inhale thoroughly, with lungs full, through the nostrils.
- Hold the breath and perform Jalandhar and Mool bandhs.
- After 5 seconds release both the bandhs and plug both the ears, using index fingers.
- Now exhale very slowly and steadily, producing humming sound like a female bee (bhramar).
- Repeat the procedure 5-8 times.

Anulom Vilom

In this alternate nostril breathing exercise, inhale through one nostril, retain the breath, then exhale through the other nostril in a ratio of 1: 4: 2. One round of Anulom vilom comprises six steps, as follows:

- Breathe in through the left nostril, while keeping the right nostril closed by thumb.
- Hold the breath, closing both the nostrils.
- Breathe out through the right nostril, keeping the left nostril closed with ring and little fingers.
- Breathe in through the right nostril, keeping the left nostril closed.
- Hold the breath, closing both the nostrils.
- Breathe out through the left nostril, keeping the right one closed with the thumb.

———::::::::———

PREKSHA MEDITATION

- Posture 156
- Mudra 156
- Recitation of Mahaprana dhwani 157
- Kayotsarga (Relaxation with self-awareness) 157
- Antaryatra (Internal trip) 158
- Shwas preksha (Perception of breathing) 158
- Sherir preksha (Perception of body) 160
- Chaitanaya kendra preksha (Perception of psychic centres) 160
- Leshya dhyana (Perception of psychic colours) 162
- Anupreksha (Contemplation) 163

Preksha Meditation

To prepare for the practice of Preksha meditation, the knowledge of postures, mudras etc. is necessary.

Posture

Either of the following postures may be adopted:

Sitting postures:

1. Padmasana (full lotus posture)
2. Ardhpadmasana (Half lotus posture)
3. Sukhasana (Simple posture)
4. Vajrasana (Diamond posture)

Standing posture: In this posture one should stand erect with the spine and neck in a straight line without any stiffness. Feet should remain 10 cm apart and parallel to each other. Arms should hang down loosely and should remain close to the body with palms open facing inward.

Mudra

Specific position of hand in sitting posture is called 'mudra'.

Gyan mudra: While sitting in either of the four above mentioned sitting postures keep the right hand on right knee while keeping left hand on left knee. Index finger should make firm contact with the thumb, making a small circle, whereas other fingers should be kept straight.

Brahma mudra: While sitting in either of the four sitting postures, bend both the arms at the elbows, keep the back of left hand on the lap and back of right hand on the top of upturned palm of left hand.

Recitation of 'Mahaprana dhwani'

- After adopting either of the postures and mudras, keep the eyes closed softly.
- Inhale deeply with lungs full, for 5-6 seconds.
- Pressing the lips together, exhale slowly without interruption, producing the sound and resonating it like buzzing of a bee, for about 10 seconds.
- Again inhale deeply and repeat the performance for at least five times.

Kayotsarga (Relaxation with self-awareness)

- After completing the recitation of **Mahaprana Dhwani**, maintain the posture and keep the spine and neck straight without any stiffness.
- Relax all the muscles of the body, making them limp.
- Concentrate your mind on each part of the body, one by one, starting with the toe of the right foot.
- Spread your conscious mind throughout all parts of every organ from the toe up to the head.
- Allow each part to relax by the process of auto-suggestion and feel that it has become relaxed.
- This way let both the feet, waist, abdomen, thorax, both the hands, neck and head including internal organs, be relaxed completely.
- Experience that the whole body is completely relaxed. Withhold this relaxed condition throughout the meditational session.

Antaryatra (Internal trip)

- Now focus your full attention on the bottom of the spinal cord, which is termed **Shakti kendra** (Centre of energy).
- Thereafter direct your attention to travel upwards along the spinal cord up to the top of the head, i.e. Gyan kendra (Centre of knowledge), and then direct it to move downward to Shakti kendra, through the same route.
- Repeat this process several times and concentrate your consciousness on the path of the trip.
- Perceive the sensations therein caused by the subtle vibrations of the flow of vital energy.
- Try to synchronise the ascending and descending movements of conscious attention with the rate of respiration, i.e. inhalation with downward movement and exhalation with upward movement.

Shwas Preksha (Perception of breathing)

Deergha shwas preksha :

- Regulate the breathing, making it slow, deep and rhythmic, along with full attention to breathing only, excluding all thoughts and sensations.
- Focus your attention on the navel and remain fully aware of the contraction and expansion of the abdominal muscles during exhalation and inhalation respectively.
- Continuously practice slow, deep and rhythmic breathing and only perceive it. Remain with deep concentration and full alertness.

- Now shift your attention from the navel and focus it inside the nostrils at the meeting point of both the nasal cavities and perceive each incoming and outgoing breath.
- Remain fully aware of each breath coming and going, and keep it slow, deep and rhythmic. Maintain the awareness of breathing while perceiving it without like and dislike.
- If any distortion occurs, due to thought, do not stop it, let it come, perceive it and then again return to the process of perception of breath.

Perception of alternate breathing :

- Regulate your breathing, making it slow, deep and rhythmic.
- Concentrate your mind inside the nostrils, and practice breathing through alternate nostrils. Inhale through the left nostril and exhale through the right one. Then inhale through right nostril and exhale through the left one.
- Repeat this process several times while keeping the breath slow, deep and rhythmic and perceiving each inhalation and exhalation with full concentration of mind in the alternate nostrils without any thought, memory and imagination.
- Perception of alternate breathing can be practised by holding the breath intermittently. With full concentration of mind inside the nostrils inhale deeply through left nostril and hold the breath inside for a few seconds (without causing any discomfort); exhale through right nostril and again hold the breath outside comfortably; then again inhale through

right nostril and hold the breath inside, exhale through left nostril and hold the breath outside. This completes one cycle of alternate breathing. This process may be repeated with the precaution that no extra pressure or pain should be taken while performing it.

Sharira Preksha (Perception of body)

The practice of the perception of body is the process in which one has to concentrate his/her mind on each part of the body, one by one and perceiving the sensations and vibrations in each part.

Starting with the big toe of the right foot, moving upwards, perceive the whole body, focusing total attention on each part of the body, till you reach the top of the head. For each organ and part of the body, one should try to penetrate maximum inside along with full attention and concentration for a few seconds.

At the end of this pratice, to perceive the body as a whole, you may stand up slowly and carefully, with the eyes remaining closed. Allow the mind to travel from toe to head and back, passing through each part/organ of the body, and continue to perceive the sensations and vibrations throughout the body. After that you can resume your sitting posture for the next step of preksha, if desired.

Chaitanya Kendra Preksha (Perception of Psychic Centers)

In the sitting, motionless and relaxed posture of the body, focus your attention on the following **Chaitanya Kendras** (Psychic centres) one by one, starting with **Shakti kendra** (Centre of energy), and feel the vibrations being produced by the flow of vital energy through these centres:

No.	Name of kendra	Corresponding gland / organ	Location
1.	Shakti kendra (Centre of energy)	Gonads	Bottom end of spinal cord
2.	Swasthya kendra (Centre of general health)	Gonads	Lower abdomen
3.	Taijasa kendra (Centre of bioelectricity)	Adrenals	Navel
4.	Ananda kendra (Centre of bliss)	Thymus	Near the heart
5.	Vishuddhi kendra (Centre of purity)	Thyroid/ parathyroid	Throat
6.	Brahma kendra (Centre of vital energy)	Organ of taste	Tongue's tip
7.	Prana kendra (Centre of vital energy)	Organ of smell	Nasal opening
8.	Chakshus kendra (Centre of vision)	Organ of sight	Eyes
9.	Apramada kendra (Centre of vigilance)	Organ of hearing	Ears
10.	Darshan kendra (Centre of intuition)	Pituitary	Middle of eyebrows
11.	Jyoti kendra (Centre of enlightenment)	Pineal	Centre of forehead
12.	Shanti kendra (Centre of peace)	Hypothalamus	Frontal part of head
13.	Gyan kendra (Centre of wisdom)	Cerebral cortex	Top of head

Leshya Dhyana (Perception of psychic colours)

Leshya dhyana is the perception of psychic colours. In the process of leshya dhyana, one should perceive a specific colour on a specific psychic centre. In leshya dhyana the following five bright colours are visualized:

1. Green colour — as of emerald
2. Blue colour — as of peacock's neck
3. Red colour — as of rising sun
4. Yellow colour — as of pure gold
5. White colour — as of full moon

The actual appearance of a particular colour at the centre is obtained only after the state of steadiness and full alertness of mind. As the steadiness of mind increases, visualizatin of a particular colour increases and ultimately the desired colour is produced.

Colours to be visualized at the respective psychic centres and the matter of intense willing and experience may be taken as follows:

No.	Psychic centre	Colour to be visualized	Intense willing
1.	Ananda kendra (Centre of bliss)	Emerald green	Freedom from psychological faults and negative attitudes
2.	Vishuddhi kendra (Centre of purity)	Peacock-neck blue	Self control of urges and impulses
3.	Darshan Kendra (Centre of intuition)	Rising sun red	Awakening of intuition: bliss
4.	Gyan kendra (Centre of wisdom) and Chakshus kendra (Centre of vision)	Golden yellow	Acuity of perception
5.	Jyoti kendra (Centre of enlightenment)	Full moon white	Tranquility

Anupreksha (Contemplation)

Practice of contemplation comprises two different categories, which are as follows:

I. To contemplate and reflect on eternal reality. This enables the practitioner to come face to face with reality.

II. To obtain attitudinal changes by the process of auto-suggestion and repeated recitation. In fact, it is the practical application of will power that the practitioner has achieved and reinforced by earlier-mentioned processes of Preksha meditation.

It is basically the concentration of thought process, in which the practitioner contemplates on an eternal or transcendental truth, which yields the realization of the truth on the level of real experience. In the other category of contemplation, the practitioner resorts to the technique of autosuggestion to cure physical sickness, mental imbalance and psychological distortions. This not only brings physical health and mental equilibrium, but also leads to development of a strong reasoning mind of the practitioner. The practitioner acquires the capability to transmute habitual negative attitude and psychological distortions and develops positive attitudes and internal harmony. In this category of exercise, concentration of mental equipment is coupled with autosuggestion. Fearlessness, amity, forbearance, transitoriness and several other characteristics and values can be contemplated by this technique.

———:::::::———

A HEALTHY ADVICE

Self-diagnosis and self-treatment is strongly denied. Expert advice/ guidance should always be sought for all diseases and disorders

SECTION III

PREKSHA-YOGIC MANAGEMENT OF COMMON DISEASES AND DISORDERS

- General precautions 166
- Headache 167
- Thyroid diseases 169
- Hypothyroidism 170
- Coronary heart disease 172
- Hypertension 174
- Asthma and bronchitis 176
- Viral rhinitis and sinusitis 179
- Tonsillitis 181
- Diarrhoea 182
- Constipation 184
- Peptic ulcer 186
- Hepatitis 188
- Obesity 191
- Diabetes 194
- Arthritis 197
- Spondylitis 200
- Herniated disc (slipped disc) 201
- Piles (haemorrhoids) 204
- Herina 205
- Menstrual abnormalities 208
- Eye problems 211
- Stress 216
- Anxiety disorder 218
- Drug addiction 219

In this section a few selected diseases, their causative factors and symptoms are discussed in brief. With the description of each disease, in the end a Preksha-yoga therapy capsule has been given to manage the disease. The capsule includes:

- Shat kriyas
- Yogic exercises
- Asanas
- Mudra and bandh
- Pranayama
- Kayotsarga (Relaxation)
- Preksha
- Anupreksha
- Dietary recommendations

To get better results one should adopt the full capsule, under the strict guidance of a qualified Preksha-yoga teacher/ instructor. The duration of various components of a capsule prescription for a particular disease should be decided by an expert.

It is worthwhile to mention that a healthy man or woman may also adopt basic exercise capsule programme to maintain the sound health and keep away the psychosomatic diseases. Such a programme is given at the end of the book.

General Precautions

1. All the exercises should be learnt well with an expert before performing them at your own. It involves ample risks if done without adequate training.
2. While performing either of the exercises no extra pain and pressure should be exerted. Learn it slowly

and then move ahead very slowly to get final posture of an exercise. If there is any problem, stop it immediately and consult the teacher.

3. If you have undergone any surgery or you are suffering from a serious chronic disease, you must take extraordinary precaution while selecting the exercises.
4. In case of pregnancy only very selected excecises are to be adopted as per advice of expert.
5. Only selected diseases have been incorporated in this book. For other diseases you should take the advice of an Preksha yoga expert.
6. Select a quiet, peaceful and open place for your exercises.
7. Wear loose and comfortable but limited clothing for your exercises.
8. Avoid closed room, bright flood light and loud music system while doing exercises.

Headache

Headache is such a common complaint that can occur for so many different reasons that its proper evaluation may be difficult. The intensity, quality and site of pain — and especially the duration of the headache and the pressure of associated neurologic symptoms — may provide clues to the underlying cause. The onset of severe headache in a previously healthy patient is more likely than chronic headache to relate to an intracranial disorder such as subarachnoid haemorrhage or meningitis. Headaches that disturb sleep, exertional headache and late-onset paroxysmal headaches are also suggestive of an underlying structural lesion, as all headaches accompanied by neurologic symptoms such as drowsiness, visual or limb problems, seizures or altered mental status. Chronic headaches are commonly due to migraine, tension or depression, but they may be related to intracranial lesions, head injury, cervical spondylosis, dental or ocular disease, temporo-mandibular joint dysfunction, sinusitis, hypertension, and a wide variety of general medical disorders.

Tension headache: Patients frequently complain of poor concentration and other vague non-specific symptoms, in addition to constant daily headaches that are often vice-like or tight in quality and may be exacerbated by emotional stress, fatigue, noise or glare. The headaches are usually generalised; may be most intense about the neck or both of the head.

Depression headache: Such headaches are frequently worse on arising in the morning and may be accompanied by other symptoms of depression. These are associated occasionally with the focus of a somatic delusional system.

Migraine headache: Migraine headache is a special type of headache that is thought to result from abnormal vascular phenomena, though the exact mechanism is unknown. It often begins with various prodromal sensations, such as nausea, loss of vision in parts of the fields of vision, visual aura or other types of sensory-hallucinations. Ordinarily the prodromal symptoms begin half an hour to an hour prior to the beginning of the headache itself.

Alcoholic headache: As many people (those who drink) have experienced, a headache usually follows an alcoholic binge. It is most likely that alcohol, because it is toxic to tissues, directly initiates the meninges and causes the cerebral pain.

Headache caused by constipation: Constipation causes headache many a time. This probably results from absorbed toxic products or from changes in the circulatory system. Indeed, constipation sometimes causes temporary loss of plasma into the wall of the gut, and the resulting poor flow of blood to the head could be the cause of the headache.

Preksha — Yoga management of headache

Shat kriyas	Kunjal Jal Neti
Yogic kriyas	For head For neck
Asanas	Surya Namaskar Pawan muktasana Sarvangasana
Kayotsarga	30 minutes at a stretch
Pranayama	Nadi shodhan Bhramari
Preksha	Perception of bright white colour at forehead
Anupreksha	To contemplate "My headache is getting subsided"
Dietary recommendations	• Simple vegetarian diet without spices • Avoid rich food, cheese, chocolate, alcohol and over-eating

Thyroid Diseases

The thyroid gland is located immediately below the larynx on either side of and anterior to the trachea. It secretes large amounts of two hormones: **thyroxin(T_4)** and **triiodothyroxine(T_3)**. These hormones have a profound effect on the metabolic rate of the body, which includes build-up and replacement of tissues, storage of energy, breakdown of tissues and utilization of the energy produced in the cells. It also secretes **calcitonin**, a hormone that is important for calcium metabolism. Complete lack of thyroid secretion usually causes the basal metabolic rate to fall to about 50 percent below normal, and extreme excesses of thyroid secretion can cause the basal metabolic rate to rise as high as 60 to 100 percent above normal. The secretion of thyroid gland is primarily controlled by thyroid-stimulating hormone secreted by the master endocrine gland, the **Pituitary gland**.

Hypothyroidism

Hypersecretion of thyroid hormone may be due to an autoimmune disesase, called *exophithalmic goitre,* also called Grave's disease. This disease is more frequent in females. One of its primary symptoms is an enlarged thyroid, called *goitre*, which may be two-three times its original size. Two other symptoms are an oedema behind the eye, which causes the eye to protrude (exophthalmos) and an abnormally high metabolic rate. The high metabolic rate produces a range of effects that generally includes higher pulse rate, high body temperature, heat intolerance, and moist flushed skin. The person loses weight and is usually full of 'nervous' energy. This condition also increases the responsiveness of the nervous system, causing the person to become irritable and exhibit tremors of the extended fingers

Hyposecretion of thyroid hormone occurs during foetal life or infancy, or during adulthood, which are known as

cretinism and **myxedema** respectively. Two outstanding clinical symptoms of the cretin are dwarfism and mental retardation. Cretin also exhibits retarded sexual development and a yellowish skin colour. Flat pads of fat develop, giving the cretin a characteristic round face and thick nose; a large, thick, protruding tongue and protruding abdomen. Cretins also have a low body temperature, slow heart rate and suffer from general lethargy. Like the cretins, the person suffering from myxedema has slow heart rate, low body temperature, sensitivity to cold, dry hair and skin, muscular weakness, general lethargy and a tendency to gain weight easily. The long-term effect of a slow heart rate may overwork the heart muscle, causing the heart to enlarge. Myxedema occurs much frequently in females than in males.

Preskha — Yoga management

Yogic exercise	Of neck
Asanas	Sarvangasana Matsyasana Viparitkarni mudra Surya Namaskar Pawan muktasana
Pranayama	Ujjayai Nadi shodhan
Kayotsarga	20 minutes
Bandh	Jalandhar bandh
Preksha	Perception of long deep breathing (Deergha shwas preksha) with blue colour on Vishuddhi kendra
Anupreksha	Contemplation for the correction of thyroid problem
Dietary recommendation	To increase the iodine intake

Coronary Heart Disease

Coronary heart disease is the commonest cause of the cardiovascular disability and death. This pathological state includes **Arteriosclerotic coronary artery disease** and **Ischaemic heart disease**.

The heart functions as the pumping station for the supply of blood to the whole body, whereas **coronary arteries**, which come out of the aorta, supply the blood and feed the heart muscles themselves. The main coronary arteries lie on the surface of the heart, and small arteries penetrate into the cardiac muscle mass. The **left coronary artery** supplies mainly the anterior part of the left ventricle, whereas the **right coronary artery** supplies most of the right ventricle as well as the posterior part of the left ventricle. The resting coronary blood flow in the human being averages approximately 225 ml per minute, which is about 4 to 5 percent of the total cardiac output. During extra work period the heart increases its cardiac output as much as four to five folds, and it pumps the blood against a higher than normal arterial pressure. Consequently the work output of the heart under severe conditions may increase as six to eight fold. The coronary blood flow also increases four to five fold to supply the extra nutrients needed by the heart.

Coronary artery disease (CAD) is a condition in which the heart muscle receives an inadequate amount of blood because of an interruption of its blood supply. Depending on the degree of interruption, symptoms can range from a mild chest pain to a full-scale heart attack. Generally, the symptoms manifest themselves when there is about a 75 percent narrowing of coronary artery lumen. The underlying causes of CAD are many and varied. Two of the principal ones are **atherosclerosis** and **coronary artery spasm**.

Atherosclerosis (sometimes called **'hardening of the arteries'**) is a situation characterized by a thickening of the arterial wall with (i) large number of smooth-muscle cells and (ii) deposits of cholesterol and other substances in the portion of the vessel wall closest to the lumen. The mechanism that initiates this thickening is not clear, but it is known that cigarette smoking, high plasma cholesterol concentration, hypertension, diabetes and several other factors increase the incidence and the severity of the atherosclerotic process. The extra muscle cells and various deposits in the wall bulge into the lumen of the vessel and increase resistance to flow. This is usually progressive, often leading ultimately to complete occlusion. Acute coronary occlusion may occur because of (i) sudden formation of blood clot on the roughened vessel surface, (ii) the breaking off of a fragment of blood clot or fatty deposit that then lodges downstream, completely blocking a smaller vessel, or (iii) a profound spasm of the vessel, smooth muscle.

Coronary artery spasm is a condition in which the smooth muscle of a coronary artery undergoes a sudden contraction, resulting in vaso-constriction. It typically occurs in individuals with atherosclerosis and may result in chest pain during rest, chest pain during exertion, heart attacks and sudden death. Although the causes of coronary artery spasm are not well known, smoking, stress and alcoholism are said to be the triggerin agents.

Preksha — Yoga management

Shat kriyas	Jal neti
Yogic exercises	Of neck and chest
Asanas	Hridyastambhasana, Pawan muktasana Vajrasana and Shashankasana
Pranayama	Nadi shodhan and Ujjayai pranayama
Kayotsarga	40 minutes, twice a day
Preksha	(i) Deergha shwas preksha (ii) Meditate with full concentration of mind on heart and coronary arteries
Anupreksha	Contemplation of fearlessness
Life style change	To adopt a stressfree habit, try to remain happy and cheerful, and to get completely away from smoking and drinking.
Dietary recommendations	• Diet should be light, avoid meat, excessive protein, milk and dairy products, oil and excessive spices. • These may be replaced with whole grains, fresh fruits and vegetables. • Overeating should be avoided. • Meal timing should be fixed.

Hypertension

Hypertension, or high blood pressure, is the most common disease affecting the heart and blood vesels. There is an agrèement at large that a blood pressure of 120/80 is normal in a healthy adult. Borderline high blood pressure is defined as diastolic pressure between 85 and 90. Mild high blood pressure is diastolic pressure between 91 and 104.

Moderate high blood pressure is diastolic pressure between 105 and 115. Severe high blood pressure is diastolic pressure of 116 or higher. Isolated systolic hypertension is systolic pressure greater than 160 in those whose diastolic pressure is less than 90.

Until recently, hypertension was diagnosed and categorised primarily based upon diastolic blood pressure readings. However, it has long been recognised that morbidity and mortality increase as both systolic and diastolic blood pressures rise, and that in individuals over age 50 the systolic blood pressure is a better predictor of complications.

In theoretical terms, hypertension could result from an increase in cardiac output or in total peripheral resistance or both. In reality, however, the major abnormality in most cases of well-established hypertension is increased total peripheral resistance, caused by abnormally reduced arteriolar lumen. For more than 95 percent of the persons with hypertension, the cause of hypertension is known, and in that condition it is called **essential hypertension** or **primary hypertension**. The remaining percentage is **secondary hypertension,** which has an identifiable underlying cause, such as kidney disease and adrenal hypersecretion.

Hypertension causes a variety of problems. One of the organs most affected is the heart. Because the left ventricle in a hypertensive person must chronically pump against an increased arterial pressure, it develops an adaptive increase in muscle mass. In the early phases of the disease this helps maintain the heart's function as a pump. With time, however, changes in the organization and properties of myocardial cells occur, and these result in diminished contractile function and heart failure. The presence of hypertension also enhances the development of atherosclerosis and heart attacks, occlusion or rupture of a cerebral blood vessel and kidney damage. Continued high blood pressure may produce a cerebral vascular accident or stroke. In such a condition severe strain is imposed on the cerebral arteries that supply the brain. This makes them weakened, which ultimately ruptures, causing brain haemorrhage.

The kidneys are another prime targets of hypertension. Continually high blood pressure causes narrowing of the lumen of the arterioles that supply to the kidney, thereby gradually reducing the blood supply. To combat this situation, kidneys secrete *renin,* which further raises the blood pressure and aggravates the problem. The reduced blood supply to the kidney may lead to death of several kidney cells.

Preksha — Yoga mangement

Shat kriyas	Jal neti and kunjal
Yogic exercises	Of neck and chest
Asanas	Tadasana, Pawan muktasana and Shashankasana
Pranayama	Chandrabhedi pranayama
Kayotsarga	40 minutes, twice a day
Preksha	Perception of body along with blue colour
Anupreksha	Contemplation of peace
Life style and dietary recommendations	• To live stress-free and peaceful life • To stop smoking, consumption of alcohol and coffee etc. • To consume less salt and fat but more potassium and calcium

Asthma and Bronchitis

Asthma is defined as a disease characterized by an increased responsiveness of the trachea and bronchi to various stimuli, and is manifested by widespread narrowing of the airway passage that changes in severity either spontaneously or as a result of treatment. It is characterized by periods of coughing, difficult breathing and wheezing. Attacks are brought on by the spasms of the smooth muscles that lie in the walls of the smaller bronchi and bronchioles, causing the passage-ways to close partially. The patient has trouble exhaling and the alveoli may remain inflated during expiration.

Usually the mucus membranes that line the respiratory passage-ways become irritated and secrete severe excessive amount of mucus that may clog the bronchi and bronchioles and worsen the attacks. About 75 percent asthma patients are found to be allergic to edible or air-borne substances. Others are sensitive to the proteins of harmless bacteria that inhabit the paranasal sinuses, nose and throat. Asthma might also have a psychosomatic origin.

Attacks of asthma are being sponsored by both physical or psychological factors. It may be triggered by emotions, environmental extremities (extreme cold exposures) and viral infections. Asthmatic attacks may also be generated and triggered in brain itself. A person who is allergic to a particular medicine may get asthmatic attack merely on looking at that medicine. Emotion generating thoughts lying in the subconscious level lead to asthmatic attack and the individuals who are unable to express their feelings may also be prone to that.

This disease is regarded primarily as a subacute inflammatory disease of airways. Multiple complex mechanisms are involved in this reversible airflow obstruction. The sensitized tissue mast cell plays a pivotal role in asthma by degranulating and releasing mediators such as histamine, bradykinin, chemotactic factors, platelet-activating factor and metabolites of arachidonic acid such as prostaglandins and leukotrienes. Neural factor may augment this response. These mediators act locally to effect broncho-constriction, cellular infiltration, platelet activation, increased vascular permeability, oedema and increased secretion of mucus. Besides mast cells, other lung cells, including eosinophils, neutrophils and lymphocytes, play important roles in the immuno-pathogenesis of airways inflammation in asthma.

Bronchitis is basically the inflammation of the bronchi and is characterized by hypertrophy and hyperplasia of seromucous glands and goblet cells lining the bronchial airways. The typical symptom of this disease is a productive cough, in which a thick green-yellowish sputum is raised. Cigarette smoking remains the most important cause of chronic bronchitis, whereas other factors that influence the development of the disease are the family history, air pollution, carbon monoxide, respiratory infections and deficient antibodies, particularly IgA antibodies.

Preksha — Yoga mangement

Shat kriya	Jal neti and kunjal
Yogic kriyas	Of respiration and chest
Asanas	Paschimottanasana, Bhujangasana, Matsyasana, Hridaya stambhasana and Naukasana
Pranayama	Suryabhedi, Anulom-Vilom and Ujjayai (all without kumbhaka)
Kayotsarga	30 minutes, twice a day
Preksha	Perception of Deergh shwas and Samvritti shwas preksha
Anupreksha	Contemplation of health of trachea and bronchi
Life-style changes	To adhere strictly with time schedule for daily routine and to avoid stay in polluted atmosphere

Viral Rhinitis and Sinusitis

Viral rhinitis

It is the 'Common Cold', whose nonspecific symptoms are present in the early phases of many diseases that affect the upper aerodigestive tract. As there are numerous serologic types of viruses, patients remain susceptible throughout life. Headache, nasal congestion, watery rhinorrhoea, sneezing and a scratchy throat accompanied by general malaise are typical in viral infections. Nasal passage usually shows reddened, oedematous mucosa and a watery discharge. The presence of purulient nasal discharge suggests bacterial infection.

Sinusitis

Secretions produced by the mucous membranes of the paranasal sinuses drain into the nasal cavity. An inflammation of the membranes due to an allergic reaction or infection is called sinusitis. If the membranes swell enough to block drainage into the nasal cavity, fluid pressure builds up in the paranasal sinuses, and a sinus headache results. Sometimes this headache is associated with swelling and tenderness over the cheek bones and forehead. Sometimes the pain becomes very severe and is accompanied by irritation in the eyes.

If the sinusitis is not managed properly, it may become a chronic disease and lasts for months and years together. During the chronic state of sinusitis, a seat of infection develops, which becomes unmanageable through conventional medical devices. This may also cause initiation of several other respiratory diseases.

Allergic rhinitis (Hay fever)

Hay fever contains the symptoms similar to those of viral rhinitis but are usually more persistent and show seasonal variation. Nasal symptoms are often accompanied by eye irritation, which causes pruritis, erythema and excessive tearing. Medical science recognises it as an allergic state that may develop from the exposure to certain allergens, found in house dust, dietary substances and pollens. Pollens are most common in spring, grasses in summer and ragweed in the fall. Dust and household units may produce year-round symptoms. Household food materials, which may contain allergens producing hay fever are chocolate, milk, bananas, strawberries etc.

The root cause of hay fever is the hypersensitivity of the individual's T-cell and B-cell immune surveillance system, which sets to start an aggressive inflammatory reaction following contact with a particular allergen.

Preksha — Yoga management

Shat kriyas	Jal neti, kapal bhati and kunjal
Yogic kriyas	Of head and neck
Asanas	Surya Namaskar, Pawan muktasana, Uttanpadasana, Simhasana, Bhujangasana, Dhanurasana and Matsyasana
Pranayama	Nadi shodhan, Suryabhedi and Bhastrika — five rounds each of 5 minutes
Kayotsarga	20 minutes daily
Preksha	Concentration of mind on nasal passages and mouth with yellow colour
Anupreksha	Contemplation of the correction of sinusitis and hay fever
Diet	• To drink plenty of water of normal temperature only • To consume light and non-mucous forming food • To avoid heavy and fatty food including sweets and fried items • To avoid consuming ice, frozen and refrigerated food materials
Life style	• To take steam inhalation • To keep the body warm • To avoid cold exposure • To stop the tobacco smoking

Tonsillitis

The tonsils are a group of small rounded organs in the pharynx. They are filled with lymphocytes and macrophages and have openings to the surface of the pharynx. Their lymphocytes respond to infectious agents that arrive by way of ingested food as well as inspired air. Basically tonsils are a multiple aggregation of large lymphatic nodules embedded in a mucous membrane. They are arranged in a ring at the junction of the oral cavity and pharynx. The single **pharyngeal tonsil** or **adenoid** is embedded in the posterior wall of the naso-pharynx. The paired **palatine tonsils** are situated in the tonsillar fossae between the pharyngopalatine and glossopalatine arches. These are the ones commonly removed during a tonsillectomy. The paired **lingual tonsils** are located at the base of the tongue.

Tonsillitis is characterised by inflammation of tonsils. They turn to become red, swollen, tender and covered with creamy waste material. This problem occurs at various intervals during childhood and adolescent period of growth, when immune system is not fully developed and the body is exposed to various organisms entering through food and air. Many a times tonsillitis is followed by serious infections leading to diseases like rheumatic heart disease, arthritis and kidney disease.

Preksha — Yoga mangement

Shat kriyas	Neti kriya and warm saline-water gargle, and kunjal as required
Yogic kriya	Of neck
Asanas	Surya Namaskar, Simhasana, Trikonasana, Matsyasana and Sarvangasana
Pranayama	Mahapranadhwani, Ujjayai and Nadishodhan

Kayotsarga	15 minutes
Preksha	Meditation and visualisation of blue colour at Vishuddhi kendra
Anupreksha	Contemplation of the relaxation of tonsils
Diet	• To avoid taking very hot or very cold food • To stop consuming sweets and fried food materials • Slightly warm liquid fruit juices to be taken frequently

Diarrhoea

Diarrhoea is a common symptom that can range in severity from an acute, self-limited annoyance to a severe, life-threatening illness. Patients may use the term **diarrhoea** to refer to increased frequency of bowel movements, increased stool liquidity, a sense of facal urgency, or facal incontinence. In the normal conditions, approximately 10 litres of fluid enters the duodenum daily, of which all about 1.5 litres are absorbed by the small instestine. The colon (large intestine) absorbs most of the remaining fluid, with only 100 ml lost in the stool. From a medical point of view, diarrhoea is defined as a stool weight of more than 250 g/24 hr. In reality, quantification of stool is necessary in the case of chronic diarrhoea.

The causes of diarrhoea are myriads. Clinically diarrhoea is of two types: acute diarrhoea and chronic diarrhoea.

Acute diarrhoea

Diarrhoea that is acute in onset and persists for less than 3 weeks is most commonly caused by infectious agents, bacterial toxins or drugs. Ingestion of improperly stored or prepared food implicates food poisoning. Exposure to unpurified water may result in infection. Recent foreign travel suggests **traveller's diarrhoea** and antibiotic administration in the preceding days results in colitis and diarrhoea. The nature of the diarrhoea helps distinguish among different infectious causes, as follows:

Non-inflammatory diarrhoea: Watery, non-blood diarrhoea associated with periumbilical cramps, bloating, nausea or vomiting suggests small bowel enteritis, caused by either toxin-producing bacterium or other agents that disrupt the normal absorption and secretory process in the small intestine.

Inflammatory diarrhoea: The presence of fever and blood diarrhoea (dysentery) indicates colonic tissue damage caused by invasion or a toxin. Because these organisms involve predominantly the colon, the diarrhoea is small in volume.

Enteric fever: A severe systemic illness, manifested initially by prolonged high fevers, prostration, confusion, respiratory symptoms followed by abdominal tenderness, diarrhoea, and a rash, is due to infection with *Salmonella typhi,* which causes bacteremia and multiorgan dysfunction.

The causes of chronic diarrhoea may be grouped as follows:

1. **Osmotic diarrhoea,** due to **lactase** deficiency.
2. **Malabsorptive diarrhoea,** due to small mucosal intestinal disease, pancreatic insufficiency, intestinal resections and intestinal bacterial overgrowth.
3. **Secretory conditions,** due to increased intestinal secretion or decreased absorption.
4. **Inflammatory conditions,** due to inflammatory bowel disease.
5. **Motility disorder,** due to abnormal intestinal motility rate.

6. **Chronic infections,** due to long-time parasitic infection.

Preksha — Yoga management:

Shat kriyas	Neti and kunjal
Yogic exercises	For abdomen
Asanas	Surya Namaskar, Pawan muktasana, Shashankasana and Bhujangasana
Pranayama	Nadi shodhan, Anulom-Vilom and Bhastrika
Bandh	Jalandhar bandh
Kayotsarga	20 minutes daily
Preksha	Samvritti shwas preksha
Anupreksha	Contemplation for correction of intestinal disorder
Diet	• To perform Bhava kriya during eating • To consume simple, fresh vegetarian food • To avoid consuming spices at all • To observe fast as per requirement

Constipation

Constipation means slow movement of faeces through the large intestine, and it is often associated with large quantities of dry, hard faeces in the descending colon that accumulate because of the long time allowed for absorption of fluid.

A frequent cause of constipation is irregular bowel habits that have developed through a life-time inhibition of the normal defecation reflexes. The new-born child is rarely constipated but part of his training in the early years of life requires that he learns to control defecation, and this control is affected by inhibiting the natural defecation reflexes. Common identifiable causes of constipation are as follows.

Poor Dietary and Behavioural Habits

The majority of the persons suffering from constipation have mild symptoms that cannot be attributed to any structural abnormalities, intestinal motility disorders or systemic disease. A careful dietary assessment reveals that most of these people do not consume adequate fiber and fluids. Ingestion of 10-12 g of fiber everyday is essential for every adult individual. At least one or two glasses of fluid should be taken with every meal. One should be encouraged to heed the **call to stool** that typically occurs after meals.

Structural Abnormalities

Colonic lesions obstruct faecal passage cause constipation.

Systemic Diseses

Various other diseases can cause constipation due to neurologic gut dysfunction, myopathies, endocrine disorders and electrolyte abnormalities.

Preksha — Yoga management

Shat kriyas	Agnisara kriya, Nauli and Basti
Yogic exercises	Of abdomen
Asanas	Surya Namaskar, Pawan muktasana, Trikon-asana, Halasana, Tadasana, Kati chakrasana, Matsyasana and Ardh matsyendrasana
Pranayama	Bhastrika with kumbhaka
Bandh	Uddiyan bandh and Maha bandh
Kayotsarga	20 minutes daily
Preksha	Deergha shwas preksha
Anupreksha	Contemplation of the correction of constipation
Diet	• To avoid starch consumption • To take light meals including fresh foods, vegetables and salads • To drink plenty of water and fruit juices • To reduce the intake of salt

Peptic Ulcer

Peptic ulcer is a crate like lesion in the wall of gastro-intestinal tract that is exposed to gastric juice. It arises when normal mucosal (a layer of gastro-intestinal tract) defensive factors are impaired or are overwhelmed by aggressive luminal factors such as acid and pepsin. Peptic ulcer occasionally develops in the lower end of oesophagus, but mostly occurs on the lesser curvature of the stomach, where they are called **gastric ulcers**, or in the first part of the duodenum, where they are called **duodenal ulcer.**

The usual basic cause of peptic ulceration is too much secretion of gastric juice in relation to the degree of protection afforded by the mucous lining of the stomach and duodenum and by the neutralization of the gastric acid by duodenal juices. All areas of gastro-intestinal (GI) tract normally exposed to gastric juice are well supplied with mucous glands, beginning with the compound mucous glands of the lower oesophagus, mucous cell coating of the stomach mucous, the mucosa neck cells of the gastric glands, the deep pyloric glands that secrete mainly mucus, and finally the glands of Brunner of the upper duodenum, which secrete a highly alkaline mucous.

In addition to the mucous protection of the mucosa, the duodenum is also protected by the alkalinity of the pancreatic secretion, which contains large quantities of sodium bicarbonate that neutralizes the hydrochloric acid of the gastric juice, thus inactivating the pepsin and thereby preventing digestion of the mucosa.

Among the factors believed to stimulate an increase in acid secretion are emotions, cigarette smoking, certain foods or medications (alcohol, coffee, aspirin), and overstimulation of the vagus (X^{th}) nerve. Ulcer occurs slightly more commonly in men than in women. Although ulcers can occur in any age group, duodenal ulcers most commonly occur between the ages of 30 and 55, whereas gastric ulcers are more common between the ages of 55 and 70. Ulcers are more common in smokers and in patients receiving non-steroidal anti-inflammatory drugs on a chronic basis. Alcohol and dietary factors do not appear to cause ulcer disease. However, the role of stress is uncertain, although it is assumed to be a significant cause.

The most common complication of peptic ulcer is bleeding. Another is perforation, erosion of the ulcer all the way through the wall of the stomach or duodenum. Perforation allows bacteria and partially digested food to pass into the peritoneal cavity, producing peritonitis. A third complication is haemorrhage. When ulcer exposes and penetrates into blood vessels, it causes a heavy and rapid blood loss, which ultimately leads a condition of shock and may prove to be fatal.

Preksha — Yoga management

Shat kriyas	Neti and laghu Shankhaprakshalan
Yogic exercises	Of abdomen
Asanas	Surya Namaskara, Pawan Muktasana, Shashankasana and Shavasana
Pranayama	Bhramari and Nadi shodhan
Kayotsarga	25 minute daily
Preksha	Perception of body with visualization of white colour
Anupreksha	Contemplation of the recovery and healing of ulcer wound
Dietary recommendations	• At the beginning to consume fruit juices and milk only • Thereafter to consume light liquid diet, khichery • To avoid completely the intake of spices, heavy food, smoking and alcohol

Hepatitis

Hepatitis is characterised by the inflammation of the liver and it can be caused by many drugs (alcohol, chemicals) and toxic agents as well as by numerous viruses, whose clinical manifestations may be quite similar. Several types of hepatitis are recognised, as mentioned below:

Hepatitis A (infectious hepatitis)

It is caused by hepatitis A virus, that may cause epidemics or sporadic cases of hepatitis. Transmission of the virus is usually by the faecal-oral route, and spread is enhanced by crowding and poor sanitation. Common source outbreaks may result from contaminated water or food. It is generally a mild disease of children and young adults, characterised by anorexia, malaise, nausea, diarrhoea, fever and chills. Eventually jaundice appears. It does not cause lasting liver damage. If managed properly, it is perfectly curable.

Hepatitis B (Serum hepatitis)

It is caused by hepatitis B virus, which is usually transmitted by inoculation of infected blood and blood products and is present in saliva, semen and vaginal secretions. Infected mothers may transmit hepatitis B virus to their neonates (newborns) at the time of delivery; the risk of chronic infection in the infant is as high as 90%. The disease may also be spread by sexual contacts. Hepatitis B virus is highly prevalent in homosexuals and intravenous drug abusers.

This virus can be present for years or even a life time and can produce cirrhosis and possibly cancer of the liver. Persons who harbour the active hepatitis B virus are at the risk of cirrhosis and also become carriers.

Hepatitis D

Hepatitis D virus is a defective RNA virus that causes hepatitis only in association with hepatitis B infection and specifically only in the presence of hepatitis surface antigen HBs Agn, and it is cleared when the latter is cleared. In terms of clinical characteristics it can infect along with hepatitis B virus and aggravate the previously existing chronic hepatitis B, or may cause acute hepatitis.

Hepatitis C

It is caused by hepatitis C virus which is a single-stranded RNA virus. It is responsible for over 90% cases of post-transfusion hepatitis and many cases of sporadic hepatitis. The risk of sexual and maternal-neonatal transmission is small and may be limited to a subset of patients with high circulating levels of hepatitis C virus RNA. In many patients the source of infection is uncertain. The incubation period averages 6-7 weeks, and clinical illness is often mild, usually asymptomatic, and characterised by waxing and waning aminotransferase elevations.

Non-A, Non-B Hepatitis (NANB)

It is a form of hepatitis that can be traced to either hepatitis A or B viruses. It is rather more similar to hepatitis B and the mode of its transfusion is often found to be blood transfusion. It causes, most of the times, liver cirrhosis and cancer.

Preksha — Yoga management

Phase - I

1. Complete rest and practice of Yoga nidra, along with Kayotsarga and Deergha shwas preksha regularly

2. To strictly avoid all such foods that inhibit liver regeneration
3. To consume plenty amount of fruit juices and papaya; and to avoid non-vegetarian food items, eggs, spices, oil, butter and ghee.

This course should be carried out for at least 8 weeks and thereafter switch on to Phase-II of therapy.

Phase - II

Shat kriyas	Kunjal kriya and Vastra dhauti
Yogic kriyas	Of chest and abdomen
Asanas	Surya Namaskar, Paschimottanasana, Trikonasana, Shashankasana and Matsyasana
Pranayama	Bhastrika, Suryabhedi, and Nadi shodhan
Mudra and bandh	Yoga mudra and Uddiyan bandh
Kayotsarga	30 minutes daily
Preksha	Meditate and visualize yellow colour on liver
Anupreksha	Contemplation of the regeneration of liver
Dietary recommendations	• To consume light food • Oil, ghee spices and non-vegetarian food should be avoided • Alcohol consumption is strictly prohibited • Fresh seasonal fruits, vegetable soups and boiled vegetables should be preferred in meals

Obesity

Obesity is one of the most common disorders in medical practice and among the most frustrating and difficult to manage. Little progress has been made in its treatment in the last 25 years, yet major changes have been understood about its causes and its implications for health.

Obesity is defined as an excess of adipose tissue. The exact criterion for how much is too much is controversial. When greater quantities of energy (in the form of food) enter the body than are expended, the body weight increases. Therefore obesity is obviously caused by excess input over energy output. Excess energy input occurs only during the development phase of obesity, and once a person has become obese, all that is required of him to remain obese is that his energy input equals his energy output. For the person to reduce, the output must be greater than the input. Indeed, studies of obese persons, once they have become obese, show that their intake of food is almost exactly the same as that of person with normal weight.

Rate of feeding is normally regulated in proportion to the nutrient stores in the body. When these stores begin to approach an optimal level in a normal person, feeding is automatically reduced to prevent overstorage. However, in many obese persons this is not rue, for feeding does not slacken until body weight is far above normal. Therefore, in effect, obesity is often caused by an abnormality of the feeding regulatory mechanism. This can result from either psychogenic factors that affect the regulation or actual abnormalities of the hypothalamus itself.

Psychogenic obesity

Studies of obese patients show that a large proportion of obesity results from psychogenic factors. Perhaps the most common psychogenic factor contributing to obesity is prevalent idea that healthy eating habits require three meals a day and that each meal must be filling. Many children are forced into this habit by over-solicitous parents, and the children continue to practice it throughout life.

Genetic Factors in Obesity

The genes can direct the degree of feeding in several different ways, including (i) a genetic abnormality of the feeding centre that sets the level of nutrient storage high or low, and (ii) abnormal hereditary psychic factors that either whet the appetite or cause the person to eat as a 'release' mechanism.

Childhood Overnutrition

The number of fat cells in the adult body is determined almost entirely by the amount of fat stored in the body during early life. The rate of formation of new fat cells is especially rapid in obese infants, and it continues at a lesser rate in obese children until adolescence. Thereafter, the number of fat cells remains almost constant throughout the life. Thus, it is believed that overfeeding children, especially in infancy and to a lesser extent during the older years of childhood, can lead to a life-time obesity.

Health Consequences of Obesity

Obesity is associated with significant increase in both morbidity and mortality. A great many disorders occur with greater frequency in obese people. The most important and common of these are hypertension, type-II diabetes mellitus, hyperlipidemia, coronary artery disease, degenerative joint disease and psychological disability. But certain cancers (colon, rectum and prostate in men; uterus, biliary tract, breast and ovary in women), thromboembolic disorders, digestive tract diseases and skin disorders are also more prevalent in the obese.

The death rate increases in proportion to the degree of obesity. Relative weights of 130% are associated with an excess mortality rate of 35% and relative weights of 150% are greater than two-fold excess death rate. Persons with 'morbid' obesity have as much as a 10-fold increase in death rate.

Preksha — Yoga management

Shat kriyas	Neti and kunjal; Shankh prakshalan (as per requirement)
Yogic exercises	Of the whole body
Asanas	Surya Namaskar, Pawan muktasana
Pranayama	Bhramari, Bhastrika and Nadi shodhana
Kayotsarga	30 minutes
Preksha	Meditate and visualize yellow colour at the centre of purity
Anupreksha	Contemplate for the balanced general metabolism
Dietary recommendations	• Fasting should be avoided • Simple vegetarian food • Meal schedule should be followed strictly • Nothing should be taken between two meals • Sugar, oil and ghee, spices and refined food items should be avoided

Diabetes

Diabetes mellitus is a heterogeneous group of diseases, which all lead to an elevation of the level of glucose in blood, often called *hyperglycemia*, and also loss of glucose in the urine. It has three basic characteristics: (i) Polyurea, inability to reabsorb water, (ii) Polyphagia, excessive eating desire, and (iii) Polydipsia, excessive thirst.

Diabetes mellitus is caused mainly by reduced rate of insulin production by the insulin-producing beta cells of the *islets of Langerhans*. Two major types of diabetes mellitus are distinguished:

(i) Type-I diabetes : Juvenile diabetes

(ii) Type-II diabetes : Maturity-onset diabetes

Type-I (Juvenile Diabetes)

In this type of diabetes the hormone *insulin* is completely or almost completely absent from the islets of langerhans and plasma, and therapy with insulin is essential. It is called insulin dependent diabetes because of compulsory periodic *insulin administration* to control the rise of blood-glucose level. It can occur at any age, though it most commonly occurs during younger age.

Type-II (Maturity-onset Diabetes)

This diabetes is much more common than type-I, representing more than 30 percent of all cases. Type-II diabetes most often occurs in people who are over 40 and overweight. Since it occurs in the later stage in life, it is termed as maturity onset diabetes. In this condition of diabetes the hormone insulin is often present in plasma at near-normal or even above-normal level, and additional insulin is not required to sustain life and to maintain normal blood-glucose level. While patients with this type of diabetes produce some, or at times even excessive, insulin in their pancreas, it either is not enough for proper function or is not being produced quickly enough to influence glucose levels in the blood effectively. This happens probably due to defects in the molecular machinery that mediates the action of insulin on its target cells. That is why this diabetes is called *non-insulin dependent diabetes mellitus.*

What Causes Diabetes?

Although the causes of diabetes are still unknown, medical science does know that certain factors contribute to its development. One factor is heredity. One may have a tendency to develop diabetes because other members of the family have it. A child of non-diabetics can become diabetic, since the disease may skip generations because of genetic coding that prevents it from appearing in every generation. Stress that affects the cells of the body seems to set the stage for diabetes in these people. One such stress is extra weight. Obesity, affecting insulin utilization, contributes to diabetes. Researchers estimate that 80 percent of the people with diabetes are also overweight at the time they are diagnosed as having diabetes.

Stresses can be emotional or physical, such as surgery or a serious infection, an accident, or emotional shock. Many medications affect the body in a stressful way. Pregnancy also places extra-stresses on the body, and diabetes is often diagnosed in pregnant women or in the women who have repeated miscarriages.

People who develop diabetes, especially Type-II, frequently also have high blood pressure; people of middle or old age are more likely to develop diabetes than younger people, and women are more likely to have diabetes than men.

As mentioned earlier, Type-I diabetes develops due to *beta cell* destruction in pancreas, which happens to be attacked by the body's own defence mechanisms (a condition of autoimmune disease) in genetically susceptible persons.

The triggering events for this autoimmune response are unknown, although viral infection is a strong cause in some cases.

Diabetes Symptoms

Type -I	Type-II
• Frequent urination	• Excess weight
• Increased thirst	• Drowsiness
• Unusual hunger	• Blurred vision
• Weight loss	• Tingling and numbness in hands and feet
• Irritability	
• Weakness and fatigue	• Skin infections
• Nausea and vomiting	• Slow healing of wounds
	• Itching

* *Source:* American Diabetic Association

Glucose concentration value chart
(mg per 100 ml of blood)

Normal		
(a)	Fasting value	65-100
(b)	Post-prandial value (2 hr after meals)	100-120
Impaired glucose tolerance*		
(a)	Fasting value	105-120
(b)	Post-prandial value (2 hr after taking gluose)	120-150
Diabetes mellitus**		
(a)	Fasting value	° 120
(b)	2 hr after taking glucose	° 180

Source: WHO

* Values are the borderline

** ° Stands for equal to or greater than

Preksha — Yoga management

Shat kriyas	Neti and kunjal
Yogic kriyas	Of abdomen and respiration
Asanas	Surya Namaskar, Pawan muktasana, Uttanpadasana, Ardha matsyendr-asana, Bhujangasana and Matsyasana
Pranayama	Bhramari and Nadi shodhan
Kayotsarga	30 minutes daily
Preksha	Meditation on pankreas
Anupreksha	Contemplation for the correction of pancreatic functions
Dietary recommendations	• Low carbohydrate, sugar-free, vegetarian diet • To avoid potatoes, rice, sugar and sugar products • Salads of leafy green vegetables and lightly boiled vegetables should be preferred • Spices, oil and ghee should be consumed in minimum quantity

Arthritis

Arthritis is a group of different diseases related with bone joints (articulations). The most common of them are rheumatoid arthritis, osteoarthritis and gouty arthritis. In all of them one or more bone joints are found to be inflammated, associated with pain and stiffness in the adjoining areas of the joint including muscles.

Rheumatoid Arthritis

It is a chronic systemic inflammatory disease of unknown cause. In this disease the body attacks its own tissues, particularly its own cartilage and linings of joints. It is characterized by inflammation of the joint, swelling, pain, and loss of function. Usually this form occurs bilaterally; if left knee is affected, the right knee may also be affected, although usually not to the same degree.

The basic symptom of rheumatoid arthritis is inflammation of the synovial membrane, followed by a sequence of changes. The membrane thickens and synovial fluid accumulates. The resulting pressure causes pain and tenderness. The membrane then produces an abnormal granulation tissue called *pannus*, which adheres to the surface of the articular cartilage. The pannus formation sometimes erodes the cartilage completely. When the cartilage is destroyed, fibrous tissue joins the exposed bone ends. The tissue ossifies and fuses the joint so that it is immovable — the ultimate crippling effect of rheumatoid arthritis.

Osteoarthritis

Osteoarthritis is the most common form of joint disease, sparing no age, race or geographic areas. Millions and millions of the people, all over the world, suffer from the effects of this condition, and 90 percent of them show radiographic features of osteoarthritis in weight-bearing joints by age 40. Symptoms of the disease increase with age. It is characterised by degeneration of cartilage and by the hypertrophy of bone at the joint margins. Inflammation is usually minimal. The cartilage slowly degenerates, and as the bone ends become exposed, small bumps, or spurs or new osseous tissues are deposited on them. These spurs decrease the space of the joint cavity and restrict joint movement. The synovial membrane is rarely destroyed, and other tissues are unaffected.

The significant distinction between osteoarthritis and rheumatoid arthritis is that the former strikes the big joints (knees, hips) first, whereas the latter strikes the small joints first.

Gouty Arthritis

During the process of nucleic acid metabolism a waste product *uric acid* is being produced. The person suffering from **gout** either produces excessive amount of uric acid or is unable to excrete the normal amount of uric acid. This results in the elevation of blood uric acid level. In due course of time the excess amount of uric acid combines with sodium and forms sodium urate crystals, which are being deposited with the kidneys and cartilages.

In *gouty arthritis* sodium urate crystals are deposited in the soft tissues of the joints. The crystals irritate the cartilage, causing inflammation.

Preksha — Yoga management

Shat kriyas	Poorna and/or laghu Shankh prakshalan (wherever necessary), kunjal and neti
Yogic exercises	Of all joints
Asanas	Pavan muktasana, Shashankasana, Bhujangasana and Dhanurasana
Pranayama	Nadi shodhan and Bhastrika
Kayotsarga	30 minutes
Preksha	Perception of long deep breathing
Anupreksha	Contemplation of the correction of joints
Dietary recommendation	• To consume wholemeal bread, rice, chapatis, millets etc. • Pulses without any spice or masala • Boiled vegetables and salad of leafy green vegetables • Fresh seasonal fruits

Spondylitis

Ankylosing spondylitis is a chronic inflammatory disease of the joints of the axial skeleton, manifested clinically by pain and progressive stiffening of the spine. The age of onset is usually the late teens or early 20s. The incidence is greater in males than in females and symptoms are more prominent in men, with ascending involvement of the spine more likely to occur.

The onset of pain is usually gradual, and is characterised by severe pain and spasm in the back of cervical region of neck, shoulders and lower spinal region, which further radiate down. Movement of neck, shoulders and back becomes very difficult and painful. It is very often associated with tension headache. As the disease advances, sysptoms progress in a cephalad direction and back motion becomes limited, with the normal lumber curve flattened and thoracic curvature exaggerated. Chest expansion is often limited.

Cervical spondylitis is characterised by muscular spasm and pain in back of neck and shoulders. It further expands into the far regions of shoulders, arms and forearms and is accompanied by needle pricking pain sensations. In the later stages movement of neck becomes restricted and arms become almost motionless because of muscular weakness. Radiographic examinations show degeneration of the vertebral column both in neck region and downward area of the spine. Such degeneration includes narrowing of the intervertebral disc space, so that the area appears worn away and unusual elongated bony projections appear. These are called *osteophytes*. The space through which blood vessels run becomes narrowed, which causes extra pressure on the vessels, reducing the blood supply to the cranial region including brain, and leading to pain.

Preksha — Yoga management

Shat kriyas	Neti kriya
Yogic exercises	Of head, neck, shoulders, chest, arms, back and waist
Asanas	Pawan muktasana, Vajrasana, Shashank-asana, Bhujangasana, Makarasana, Dhanurasana and Matsyendrasana
Pranayama	Nadi shodhan
Kayotsarga	30 minutes
Preksha	Perception of deep breathing
Anupreksha	Contemplation of the correction of vertebral column abnormality
Dietary recommendations	• To consume plenty of protein and boiled vegetables • To increase the intake of fresh seasonal fruits

Herniated Disc *(Slipped disc)*

The vertebral column (spine), together with sternum and ribs, constitutes the skeleton of the trunk of the body. The vertebral column makes up about two-fifths of the total height of the body and is composed of a series of bones called vertebrae.

The adult vertebral column typically contains 26 vertebrae. These are distributed as: *7 cervial vertebrae* (in the neck region); *12 thorasic vertebrae* (chest region); *5 lumbar* vertebrae (supporting the lower back); *5 sacral vertebrae* (fused together into one bone called sacrum); and usually *4 coccygeal vertebrae* (fused into one or two bones called coccyx). Prior to the fusion of the sacral and coccygeal vertebrae, the total number of vertebrae is 33.

Between adjacent vertebrae from the first vertebra to the sacrum are fibrocartilaginous *intervertebral discs*. Each disc is composed of an outer fibrous ring consisting of fibrocartilage, called the *annulus fibrosus* and an inner soft, pulpy, highly elastic structure, called *nucleus pulposus*. The discs form strong joints, permit various movements of the vertebral column and absorb vertebral shock.

The intervertebral discs are subject to compressional forces while performing the function of shock absorbers. The discs between the fourth and fifth lumbar vertebrae and between the fifth lumbar vertebra and sacrum usually are subject to more forces than other discs. If the anterior and posterior ligaments of the discs become injured or weakened, the pressure developed in the nucleus pulposus may be great enough to rupture the surrounding fibro-cartilage. If this happens, the nucleus pulposus may protrude (herniate) posteriorly or into one of the adjacent vertebral bodies. This state is called *herniated disc* or *slipped disc*.

Most often the nucleus pulposus slips posteriorly towards the spinal cord and spinal nerve. This movement exerts pressure on the spinal nerves, causing considerable, sometimes very acute, pain. When intra-abdominal pressure is increased by coughing, sneezing or other movement, symptoms are aggravated, and cervical muscle spasm may often occur. Neurologic abnormalities may include decreased reflexes of the deep tendons of the biceps and triceps and decreased sensation and muscle atrophy or weakness in the forearm or hand.

Preksha — Yoga management

Initially the patients should be made immobilized without any delay on a hard bed. For fast recovery and healing complete bed rest is compulsory for a few days. Complete immobilization of spine is the safest and quickest route of healing and recovery. The duration of immobilization required depends upon the degree of injury. In the later stage preksha-yoga therapy should be applied, which promotes the recovery.

Shat kriyas	Jal neti
Yogic exercises	Of the spine (without any undue pressure)
Asanas	Mostly backward bending asanas — Makarasana; Sleeping in Advasana and Jyesti Asana — in the initial stage In the later stage — Uttanpadasana, Pawanmuktasana, Shalbhasana, Bhujangasana and Suptavajrasana
Pranayam	Anulom-Vilom and Nadi shodhan
Kayotsarga	45 minutes — thrice a day
Preksha	Perception of whole vertebral column
Anupreksha	Contemplation for correction of the injured disc
Dietary recommendations	• In the begining semiliquid diet should be taken • Khicheri and vegetable soup should be taken in the meals. Thereafter rice, pulses, boiled vegetables and wholemeal bread may be taken as the condition improves • Spices and non-vegetarion food items should not be taken

Piles *(Haemorrhoids)*

In people with weak venous valves, gravity forces large quantities of blood back down into distal parts of the vein. This pressure overloads the vein and pushes its wall outward. After repeated overloading, the walls lose their elasticity and become stretched and flabby. Such dilated and tortuous veins, caused by incompetent valves, are called **varicose veins**. These may be due to heredity, mechanical factors (prolonged standing and pregnancy), or ageing. Because a varicosed wall is not able to exert a firm resistance against the blood, the blood tends to accumulate in the pouched-out area of the vein, causing it to swell and forcing the fluid into the surrounding tissue.

Varicosity of the rectal veins is known as haemorrhoid (piles). It develops when the viens are put under pressure and become engorged with blood. If the pressure continues, the wall of the vein stretches. Such a distended vessel oozes blood, and bleeding or itching are usually the first signs that a pile has developed. Stretching of a vein also favours clot formation, further aggravating the swelling and pain. Initially contained within the anus (first degree) they gradually enlarge until they prolapse or get extended outward on defecation (second degree) and finally remain prolapsed through the anal orifice (third degree). One particular reason of piles is constipation.

Preksha — Yoga management

Yogic exercises	Of waist, legs and thighs
Asanas	Sarvangasana, Shirshasana, Tadasana, Padahastasana, Surya Namaskar, Matsyasana and Pawan muktasana
Bandh	Mool bandh

Pranayama	Nadi shodhan and Bhastrika
Kayotsarga	20 minutes daily
Preksha	Perception of gastro-intestinal tract, particularly large intestine, rectum and anus
Anupreksha	Contemplation for strengthening of rectal muscles and veins
Dietary recommendations	• Unnecessary standing should be avoided • While relaxing, try to keep the legs stretched with full rest • During pregnancy lie down by the side • To avoid strictly the spicy and fried food • To consume light and easily digestiable food items

Hernia

Hernia is the protrusion of an organ or part of an organ through a membrane or cavity wall, usually the abdominal cavity. It happens due to natural weakness of the muscles holding the organs in their original positions. It occurs both in males and females. Most commonly occurring hernias are of 3 types.

Types of Hernia

Inguinal hernia: In this type of hernia, in the groin region the testes descends into the scrotum through the narrow passage of inguinal canal. Most of the times this occurs before birth. Due to pushing down of the hernial contents into the scrotum it enlarges and becomes difficult to distinguish from the swelling of the testes or scrotum, which occurs in the condition of hydrocoele. This is most common external hernia, covering the total of 70% and is very common in men.

Umbilical hernia: This is another commonly occurring hernia, accounting for 8-10%, mostly coccurs at birth or in infancy. It may also occur in an obese person or in a person with weak abdomen in the middle age. In this hernia, the hernial sac bulges out through the umbilicus, which is the place of weak abdominal muscle.

Femoral hernia: This type of hernia is found mostly in women and it accounts for 20% of the hernias. In this the abdominal contents move into the front of the thigh through an opening which carries the femoral artery into the leg. This artery supplies the blood to the leg.

Causative Factors

Several factors are responsible for the pathological state of hernia, which may be classified as follows:

(i) Congenital weakness or the developmental defect in the abdominal muscles or ligaments, which produces hernia in the early childhood.

(ii) In the young men or women a sudden jerk while lifting any heavy item without proper precaution may result in tearing the muscles and ligaments, which ultimately produces hernia.

(iii) In the situation where the intra-abdominal pressure is elevated, it may cause hernia. In the old age, due to enlarged prostate, obstruction in urine passage; continuous coughing in smokers; and strainful defecation due to constipation are few examples that produce hernia due to raised intra-abdominal pressure.

(iv) Sedentary life style, lack of adequate physical exercise, causing flabbiness of the abdominal muscles, obesity and habitual overeating may also cause hernia. In such conditions abdominal wall loses its tone and abdominal organs begin to sag. The whole abdomen protrudes markedly.

(v) In the women pregnancy and child birth also cause hernia due to increased abdominal pressure in these conditions.

Preksha — Yoga management

Shat kriyas	Neti kriya, Laghu Shankh Prakshalan once a week (as required)
Yogic exercises	Of thorax, abdomen, waist and legs
Asanas	Pawan muktasana, Uttanpadasana, Sarvangasana, Paschimottanasana, Matsyasana, Vajrasana, Shashank-asana, Ushtrasana
Mudra and bandh	Ashwini mudra, Vajroli mudra, Mool bandh
Pranayama	Bhramari; Bhastrika with antar kumbhak; Anulom-Viloma without kumbhak
Kayostsarya	30 minutes daily
Preksha	Perception of abdominal muscles, intestine, rectum, rectal muscles and anal canal
Anupreksha	Contemplation for strengthening of abdominal muscles

Menstrual Abnormalities

The normal reproductive years of a women are characterised by monthly rhythmic changes in the rates of secretion of female hormones and corresponding changes in the sexual organs themselves. The rhythmic pattern is called the **female sexual cycle** or **Menstrual cycle**. The duration of the cycle averages 28 days. It may be as short as 20 days or as long as 45 days even in completely normal women, though abnormal cycle length is occasionally associated with decreased fertility. The two significant results of the female sexual cycle are: first, only a single mature ovum is normally released from the ovaries each month, so that only a single foetus can begin to grow at a time; second, the uterine endometrium is prepared for implantation of the fertilized ovum at the required time of the month.

The menstruation reflects not only the health of the uterus but also the health of the endocrine glands that control it, i.e. the ovaries and the pituitarry gland. The disorders of the female reproductive system are frequently involved in the menstrual disorders. Some of them are:

Amenorrhoea

This means without monthly flow, i.e. the absence of menstruation. If a woman has never menstruated, the condition is called **primary amenorrhoea**. This can be caused by endocrine disorders, most often in the pituitary gland and hypothalamus or by genetically caused abnormal development of the ovaries or uterus. **Secondary amenorrhoea**, the skipping of one or more periods, is commonly experienced by women at some time during their life. Changes in body weight, either gains or losses, often cause amenorrhoea. Obesity may disturb ovarian function, and similarly the extreme weight loss that characterises anorexia nervosa often leads to a suspension of menstrual flow. When amenorrhoea is not related with the changes in body weight, its causative factor may be the deficiencies of pituitary and ovarian hormone. Amenorrhoea may also be caused by continuous involvement in rigorous atheletic training.

Dysmenorrhoea

It refers to pain associated with menstruation and the term is usually reserved to describe an individual with menstrual symptoms that are severe enough to prevent her from functioning normally for one or more days each month. Primary dysmenorrhoea is painful menstruation with no detectable organic disease. The pain in this condition is thought to result from uterine contractions, probably associated with uterine muscle ischaemia and prostaglandins produced by the uterus. Prostaglandins are known to stimulate uterine contractions, but they cannot do so in the presence of high levels of progesterone (a hormone secreted by ovary). Progesterone levels are high during the last half of the menstrual cycle, and during this time prostaglandins are apparently inhibited by progesterone from producing uterine contractions. However, in the absence of pregnancy progesterone levels drop rapidly and prostaglandin production increases. This causes the uterus to contract and slough off its lining, which may result in dysmenorrhoea. In addition to pain, other signs and symptoms may include headache, nausea, diarrhoea or constipation and increased urinary frequency. Secondary dysmenorrhoea is painful menstruation that is frequently associated with a pelvic pathology. In some cases it is caused by uterine tumours, ovarian cysts, pelvic inflammatory disease, endometriosis and intrauterine devices.

Abnormal Uterine Bleeding

This refers to mestruation of excessive duration or excessive amount, diminished menstrual flow, too frequent menstruation, intermenstrual bleeding and post-menstrual bleeding. The causative factors for all such conditions may be the disordered hormonal regulation, emotional imbalance and any tumour in the uterus.

Premenstrual Syndrome

It is a term usually refers to severe physical and emotional distress occurring in the post-evaluatory phase of the menstrual cycle and sometimes overlapping with menstruation. Signs and symptoms usually increase in severity until the onset of menstruation and then dramatically disappear. Among the signs and symptoms are oedema, weight gain, breast swelling and tenderness, abdominal distension, backache, joint pain, constipation, skin eruptions, fatigue and lethargy, greater need for sleep, depression or anxiety, irrtibility, headache, poor coordination and clumsiness, and craving for sweet or salty foods. Although premenstrual syndrome is related to the cyclic production of ovarian hormones, its symptoms are not directly due to the changes in these hormones' profile, and the basic cause of this state is not known.

Preksha — Yoga management

Shat kriyas	Neti — daily Kunjal and Laghu Shankh prakshalan — thrice a week
Yogic kriyas	Of abdomen and waist
Asanas	Surya Namaskar Ushtrasana, Shashankasana, Supta Vajrasana, Vajrasana, Bhujangasana, Shalbhasana, Dhanurasana, Sarvangasana, Halasana, Paschimottanasana, Matsy-asana, Pad hastasana and Tadasana
Pranayama	Nadi shodhan, Ujjayai and Bhramari
Mudra and bandh	Vipareet karni and Ashwini mudra Mool bandh
Kayotsarga	30 minutes daily
Preksha	Perception of body
Anupreksha	Contemplation for strengthening the reproductive organs
Dietary recommendations	• To consume wholesome vegetarian food • Excess oil and ghee should not be taken • Light food on the pattern of "little less then required" should be taken

Eye Problems

The eye is optically equivalent to the usual photographic camera, for it has a lens system, a variable aperture system, and a retina that corresponds to the film. The lens system of the eye is composed of (i) the interface between air and the anterior surface of the cornea, (ii) the interface between the posterior surface of the cornea and the aqueous humor, (iii) the interface between aqueous humor and the anterior surface of the lens, and (iv) the interface between the posterior surface of the lens and the vitreous humor. The difference between the refractive indices on the two sides of each surface is one of the factors that determine the focusing strength of each surface. In exactly the same manner that a glass lens can focus an image on a sheet of paper, the lens system of the eye can also focus an image on the retina. The image is inverted, and reversed with respect to the object. However, the mind perceives the object in the upright position despite the upside-down orientation of the retina because the brain is trained to consider an inverted image as the normal.

The formation of an image on the retina requires four basic processes, all concerned with focusing light rays: (i) refraction of light rays, (ii) accommodation of the lens, (iii) constriction of the pupil, and (iv) convergence of the eyes. Accommodation and pupil size are functions of the smooth muscle cells of the ciliary muscle and the dilator and constrictor muscles of the iris. They are termed **intrinsic eye muscles**, since they are inside the eyeball. Convergence is a function of the voluntary muscles attached to the outside of the eyeball called the **extrinsic eye muscles**.

The ciliary muscle is controlled almost entirely by the parasympathetic nerves. Stimulation of the parasympathetic fibres to the eye contracts the ciliary muscle, which in turn relaxes the ligaments of the lens and increases its refractive power. With an increased refractive power, the eye is more capable of focusing on objects that are nearer to it than the eye with less refractive power. Consequently, as a distant object moves toward the eye, the number of parasympathetic impulses impinging on the ciliary muscle must be progressively inereased for the eye to keep the object in focus.

Presbyopia

As a person grows older, his lens loses its elastic nature and becomes a relatively solid mass, probably because of progressive denaturation of the proteins. Therefore the ability of the lens to assume a spherical shape progressively decreases, and the power of accommodation decreases, from approximately 14 diopters shortly after birth to approximately 2 diopters at the age of 45 to 50. Thereafter, the lens of the eye may be considered to be almost totally non-accommodating, which condition is known as *presbyopia*.

Hypermetropia

A normal eye is considered to be 'emmetropic', when the ciliary muscle is completely relaxed, parallel light rays from distant objects are in sharp focus on the retina. **Hypermetropia**, also known as **'far-sightedness'**, is due either to an eyeball that is too short or to a lens system that is too weak when the ciliary muscle is completely relaxed. In this condition, parallel light rays are not bent sufficiently by the lens system to come to a focus by the time they reach the retina. In order to overcome this abnormality, the ciliary muscle must contract to increase the strength of the lens. Therefore in old age, when the lens becomes presbyopic, the far-sighted person often is not able to accommodate his lens sufficiently to focus even distant objects, much less to focus near objects.

Myopia

In myopia, or **'near-sightedness'**, even when the ciliary muscle is completely relaxed, the strength of the lens is still enough so that light rays coming from distant objects are focused in front of the retina. This is usually due to too long an eyeball, but it can occasionally result from too much power of the lens system of the eye.

Cataract

A cataract is a clouding of the lens or its capsule so that it becomes opaque or milky white. The two basic processes involved in cataract formation are the breakdown of the normal lens protein and an influx of water into the lens. As a result, the light from an object, which normally passes directly through the lens to produce a sharp image, produces only a degraded image. If the cataract is severe enough, no image at all is produced. This problem is associated with ageing, but may also be caused by injury, exposure to radiation and certain medications.

Glaucoma

It is a most common cause of blindness, especially in the elderly. In fact, it is a group of disorder characterised by an abnormally high intraocular pressure owing to a build up of aqueous humor inside the eyeball. This aqueous humor does not return into the blood-stream and accumulates there. By compresing the lens into the vitreous body, it puts pressure on the neurons of the retina, resulting in degeneration of the optic disc, visual field defects and blindness.

Nightblindness

Nightblindness occurs in severe vitamin A deficiency. When the total quantity of vitamin A in the blood becomes greatly reduced, the quantities of vitamin A, retinal and rhodopsin in the rods, as well as the colour photosensitive chemicals in the cones, are all depressed, thus decreasing the sensitivities of the rods and cones. This condition is called nightblindness because at night the amount of available light is far too little to permit adequate vision, though in daylight, sufficient light is available to excite the rods and cones despite their reduction in photochemical substances.

Preksha — Yoga management

Shatkriyes	Jal neti
Special yogic exercises	• Of head and neck • **Palming** — for local relaxation and strengthening of eye muslces • **Candle gazing** — for relaxation of eye muscles and steadying the mind • **Fucusing exercises** (i) Shoulder gazing (ii) Centre gazing (iii) Up-and-down gazing All these exercises are to train eye muscles for quicker adjustment capacity and strength • **Water cleansing** — Take a wide-mouthed bowel, full of clean and cold water. Keep this pot on a table of shoulder height. Now tilt the head downward putting the right eye in the water with eyelid open. Roll the eyeball around in the same condition for a few seconds. Repeat the process with left eye also. Repeat the exercise four-five times a day.
Asanas	Simhasana, Sarvangasana, Bhujangasana, Vajrasana, Ushtrasana, Matsyasana
Pranayama	Nadi shodhan and sheetali
Kayotsarga	30 minutes — thrice a day
Preksha	Perception of long-deep breathing with the concentration on eyes along with green colour
Anupreksha	Contemplation for strengthening the eye muscles
Dietary recommendation	• To consume light vegetarian diet, providing maximum quantity of vitamin A • To avoid chilli, spicy and stimulatory food items • To avoid going in strong sunlight, flood light and reading in inappropriate light intensity

Stress

Stress, the overused word, has found a firm place in our new age vocabulary just as fast food, junk, bond or software packages have. So debased by misuse, it generates only negativity in most people's minds.

Stress exists when the adaptive capacity of the individual is overwhelmed by events. Opinion differs about what events are most apt to produce stress reactions. The causes of stress are different at different ages. For example, in young adulthood, the sources of stress are found in marriages or parent-child relationship, the employment relationship, and the struggle to achieve the desired goal and career; in the middle age group, the focus shifts to changing spousal relationships, problems with ageing parents, professional problems, social problems and problems related to young adult offsprings who are encountering stressful situations; in old age concerns for the loss of physical capacity and isolation as well as loneliness after retirement from active life.

Stress results from an individual's appraisal of a demand as being greater than his actual or perceived ability to deal with it. The stress is normally being experienced from the following three sources:

From environment: A person is bombarded with demands to adjust constantly to time and relationship pressures, crowding noise, weather etc.

From body physiology: It could be adolescence, menopause, ageing, illness, accidents or sleep disturbances.

From self-appraisal: It comes in terms of interpretation, perception and level of demand.

The intensity level of stress is determined by the degree of imbalance between demand and coping skills. In other words, mastery of the mind gives the skill to solve problems at work. These skills change the attitude to health and bring fulfilment in the individual's life.

An individual may react to stress by becoming anxious or depressed, by developing a physical symptom, by running away, by having a drink or starting an affair, or in limitless other ways. Common subjective responses are fear, rage, guilt and shame. Acute and reactivated stress may be manifested by restlessness, irritability, fatigue, increased startle reaction, and a feeling of tension. Inability to concentrate, sleep disturbances and somatic pre-occupations often lead to self-medication, most commonly with alcohol or other neural depressants.

When an individual responds to a threatening situation, several physiological changes take place in the body, summarised as the **fight-n-flight reaction.** The problem is first assessed by the cerebral cortex, the thinking part of the brain, which then sends a signal to the hypothalamus, the switch for a stress response, and then on to the autonomic nervous system (ANS). Thereafter sympathetic part of the ANS releases an orchestra of specific chemicals. Digestion slows down, sending blood to the brain and muscles, breathing becomes faster, the heart beat steps up and perspiration increases to cool the body under stress. Sugar and fats are pumped to increase energy production to provide unusual strength and endurance during an emergency. At the same time adrenal gland (an endocrine gland) secretes cortisols, which inhibit digestion, growth, inflammatory responses and tissue repair. In other words, the same responses that keep on going begin to close down. As the brain switches off the panic signals, the chemicals are metabolised and body returns to normal. However, if stress is recurrent or body fails to adopt, disabling illness results.

It is pertinent to mention here that parasympathetic part of autonomic nervous system, which often acts as a maintenance system and secretes chemicals (neurotransmitters), affects the body in exactly the opposite way, thereby effecting a balance. However, it works at a subconscious level and consequently researches have shown that yogic stress management techniques can stimulate the sympathetic nervous system and thereby convert the fight-n-flight response to a stay-n-play response.

Preksha — Yoga management

Shat kriyas	Kunjal and Jal neti
Yogic exercises	Of the whole body
Asanas	Tadasana, Naukasana, Trikonasana, Bhujangasana, Halasana, Vajrasana
Pranayama	Bhastrika and Anulom Vilom
Kayotsarga	Supta kayotsarga (40 minutes) daily
Preksha	Perception of deep breathing and body, along with white colour
Anupreksha	Contemplation of friendship and forebearance
Yogic life-style	To strictly follow the principles of yogic life style.

Anxiety Disorder

Stress, fear and anxiety all tend to be interactive. The principal components of anxiety are *psychologic* (tension, fears, difficulty in concentration, apprehension) and *somatic* (tachycardia, hyperventilation, palpitation, tremor, sweating). Other organ systems, e.g. gastrointestinal, may be involved in multiple-system complaints. Fatigue and sleep disorders are common. Sympathomimetic symptoms of anxiety are both a response to a central nervous system state and a reinforcement of further anxiety. Anxiety can become self-generating, since the symptoms reinforce the reaction, causing it to become spiral.

Anxiety may be free-floating, resulting in acute anxiety attacks, occasionally becoming chronic. When one or several defense mechanisms are functioning the consequences are well-known problems such as phobias, conversion reactions, dissociative states, obsessions and compulsions.

Preksha — Yoga management

Shat kriyas	Kunjal and Jal neti
Yogic exercises	Of the whole body
Asanas	Shashankasana, Sarvangasana, Matsyasana, Padmasana, Bhujang-asana, Shalbhasana
Pranayama	Anulom-Vilom and Ujjayai
Kayotsarga	50 minutes daily at a stretch
Preksha	Perception of body along with white colour
Anupreksha	Contemplation of power and self-confidence
Dictory recommendations	To take sattvic food only

Drug Addiction

The psychoactive drugs or street drugs are being taken in a deliberate attempt to elevate mood (euphorigens) and produce unusual state of consciousness up to the state of hallucination. All these drugs exert their actions directly or indirectly by altering the normal functions of neurons.

Tolerance to a drug occurs when increasing doses of that drug are required to achieve effects that initially occurred in response to a smaller dose, that is it takes more drug to do the same job.

If the consumption of drug goes on along with tolerance, it culminates in **drug dependence** or **drug addiction**. Drug dependency is a function of the amount of drug used and the duration of usage. Alcohol, opioids, LSD, marijuana, cocaine, heroin, caffeine and nicotine are a few important agents that are being taken by drug users.

There is accumulating evidence that an impairment syndrome exists in drug users. It is believed that drug use produces damaged neurotransmitter receptor sites, causing **'kindling' effects** — repeated stimulation of the brain. These effects may be manifested as mood swings, panic, psychosis and occasionally overt seizure activity. The imbalance also results in personal non-productivity, frequent job changes, marital problems, negative behavioural changes and generally erratic behaviour, which in turn make the personal and family life the hell.

Preksha — Yoga management

Yogic exercises	Of the whole body
Asanas	Tadasana, Trikonasana, Halasana, Nauk-asana, Vajrasana, Bhujangasana, Shashankasana and Sarvangasana
Pranayama	Ujjayai and Supta bhastrika
Kayotsarga	30 minutes — twice a day
Preksha	Visualization of green colour at Darshan kendra
Anupreksha	Contemplation of drug de-addiction
Yoga nidra	Exclusively for drug addicts

REFERENCES

1. Acharya Mahaprajna (1994): **Preksha Dhyana: Theory and Practice**
(Muni Mahendra Kumar, Editor)
Jain Vishva Bharati, Ladnun, Rajasthan (India)

2. Alain (1964): **Yoga for Perfect health**
Thomsons Publishers Ltd., London.

3. Anantharaman, T. R. (1996): **Ancient Yoga and Modern Science**
Published by Prof. B. Chandel for PHISPC, Nirman Vihar, Delhi.

4. Dalal, N. (1951): **Yoga for Rejuvenation**
Orient Longman Limited, Hyderabad.

5. Eliade, Mircea (1969): **Yoga, Immortality and Freedom**
Routledge and Kagaun Paul Ltd., London.

6. Garde, R.K. (1984): **Yoga Therapy - Principles and Practice.**
D.B. Taraporevala Sons and Co. Pvt. Ltd., Bombay.

7. Iyengar, B.K.S. (1968): **Light on Yoga (Yoga Dipika)**
George Allen and Unwin Ltd., London.

8. Iyengar, B.K.S. (1992): **Light on Yoga**
INDUS, an Imprint of Harper Collins Publishers India Pvt. Ltd., New Delhi.

9. Iyengar, B.K.S. (1993): **Light on Pranayama**
Harper Collins Publishers, New Delhi.

10. Swami Kuvalyananda (1993): **Asanas**
Kaivalyadhama, Lonavala, Maharashtra.

11. Mc Donald, K. (1977): **How to Meditate**
Wisdom Publishers, Boston, USA; and Timeless Books (Pub.), Delhi.

12. Mehta, R. (1981): **The Science of Meditation**
Motilal Banarasidas, Delhi.

13. Nagrathna, R, Nagendra, R. and Monro, R. (1990): **Yoga for Common Ailments**
Gaia Books Limited, London

14. Niranjanananda, Paramhamsa (1977): **Yoga Dharshan**
Shri Panchdashnam Paramhamsa Alakh Bara, Bihar.

15. Pranavananda, Yogi (1992): **Pure Yoga**
Motilal Banarsidas Publishers Pvt. Ltd., Delhi.

16. Ross, Karen (1973): **The Manual of Yoga**
W. Foulshan and Co. Ltd., England.

17. Sadhu, Mouni (1967): **Meditation**
George Allen and Unwin Ltd., London.

18. Sampurnananda (1990): **Yogadarshana**
Uttar Pradesh Hindi Sansthan, Luckhnow.

19. Saraswati, Swami Karmanand (1968): **Yogic Management of Common Diseases**
Bihar School of Yoga, Munger, Bihar.

20. Saraswati, Swami Muktibodhananda (1977): **Hatha Yoga**
Bihar School of Yoga, Munger, Bihar.

21. Saraswati, Swami Satyananda (1977): **Asana, Pranayama, Mudra and Bandha**
Bihar School of Yoga, Munger, Bihar

22. Van Lysebeth, Andre (1968): **Yoga Self Taught**
(Translator - Carola Congreve):
George Allen and Unwin Ltd., London.

23. Yesudian, S. and Haich, E. (1966): **Yoga and Health**
Unwin Books, London.

———— :::::::: ————

ANNEXURE I

DAILY PREKSHA - YOGA PROGRAMME FOR GENERAL HEALTH

The seven sets of Preksha-Yoga programme are given hereunder for a common man. These should be followed in sequence starting with no. 1 onward by practising each set for at least 15 days.

First set:

- Surya Namaskar (Sun salutation)
- Yogic exercises (For whole body)
- Asanas —
  * Uttanpadasana
  * Shalbhasana
  * Simhasana
  * Tadasana
- Kayotsarga
- Pranayama
- Preksha meditation —
  * Kayotsarga
  * Perception of deep breathing
  * Perception of psychic centre (Centre of enlightenment)

Second set:

- Surya Namaskar
- Yogic exercises (as in first set)
- Asanas —
  * Pawan muktasana
  * Dhanurasana
  * Gomukhasana
  * Trikonasana

- Kayotsarga
- Pranayama
- Preksha meditation (as in first set)

Third set:

- Surya Namaskar
- Yogic exercises (as in first set)
- Asanas — * Sarvangasana
  * Bhujangasana
  * Janushirasana
  * Madhyapadshirasana
- Kayotsarga
- Pranayama
- Preksha meditation (as in first set)

Fourth set:

- Surya Namaskar
- Yogic exercises (as in first set)
- Asanas — * Halasana
  * Matsyasana
  * Paschimottanasana
  * Mahaveerasana
- Kayotsarga
- Pranayama
- Preksha meditation (as in first set)

Fifth set:

- Surya Namaskar
- Yogic exercises (as in first set)

- Asanas — * Karna peedasana
  * Supta Vajrasana
  * Ardha Matsyendrasana
- Kayotsarga
- Pranayama
- Preksha meditation (as in first set)

Sixth set:

- Surya Namaskar
- Yogic exercises (as in first set)
- Asanas — * Naukasana
  * Ushtrasana
  * Natarajasana
  * Hridaya stambhasana
- Kayotsarga
- Pranayama
- Preksha meditation (as in 1st set)

Seventh set:

- Surya Namaskar
- Yogic exercises (as in first set)
- Asanas — * Makarasana
  * Sarpasana
  * Hansasana
  * Uddiyan
- Kayotsarga
- Pranayama
- Preksha meditation

Note:

(1) The daily practice of Pranayama should be as follows:

(a) In winter season — (i) Surya bhedi
(ii) Ujjayai along with Jalandhar bandh

(b) In summer season— (i) Chandra bhedi
(ii) Sheetli
(iii) Sheetkari

(c) In other seasons or any other time
(i) Deergha shwas
(ii) Bhramari
(iii) Anulom - Vilom

(2) The practice of Preksha meditation should be carried out for long time and then can be changed as per guidance of Preksha Instructor.

(3) One of the above-mentioned seven sets should be carried out for at least 15 days before shifting to the next one.

———:::::::::———